Dancing

Collection of Hospice Stories

Psalm 91:11

Karen Farr, R.N.

Karen Farr RN

Luna —
Always Know you
are surrounded by
angels. May God
always be your strength
and Jesus your Lord.
I love you (mimi)
Karen

Dancing with Angels
Copyright © 2015
Karen Farr

Table of Contents

PREFACE

Hospice has various meanings when the word 'hospice' is first heard. Some think of it as a death sentence, while others think of a support system that allows one to experience death in their own home.

Ultimately, we will all need Hospice.

Karen Farr has written a book that allows medical professionals an opportunity to prepare to enter the field of hospice. The book provides insights for a potential hospice patient, family, caregiver, or interested person. It provides pathways to understand what hospice is and does. There are vignettes that tell the story of hospice in a way that encourages by sharing emotions related to the dying process.

In summary, the book allows readers to experience hospice as a support during a difficult time.

Randy Denham, M.S.W., M.F.C.C.

Karen's authentic account of what it is to enter the life of a terminally ill patient, who's hope is to have a sensitive hospice/palliative trained nurse as their primary case manager, will undoubtedly reach the interest of most people. For sure, Karen was called to the holiest of nursing service.

Kate Shirley, R.N.

INTRODUCTION

Dancing with Angels shares ten hospice experiences. These fictitious stories draw on events from Karen's ten years as a hospice nurse. She chooses settings and events that emphasize how hospice functions under the federal guidelines.

Red Knitted Slippers: A financially strapped Viet Nam Vet dies in his brother's home.

Heaven, I've Been There: A single mother with an 'out of body' experience has no fear of dying.

Bagels and Lox: A grandmother lives one week in her son's home after experiencing a massive stroke.

Get on Board: A grandfather has concern about his grandchildren's spirituality.

Orange Bucket: A contractor attempts all holistic and known medical interventions to cure cancer.

I Found My Lost Daughter: A Korean War vet finds a daughter born out of wedlock.

Where's Ernie? A father with Alzheimer ends his ten year journey confused in a skilled nursing facility.

I Want Chocolate at my Memorial: Hospice care extends the life of a ninety-four year old chocoholic grandmother.

Queen Victoria: A widow without family wrestles with her self-image.

B-17 Bomber's Final Flight: A World War II Veteran struggles with his wife's difficulties in accepting his death.

Each story shares a hospice journey and how different people faced the reality of death.

Hospice does not promise to add or subtract days to life. These stories show how some patients lived longer and more comfortably when hospice controlled their symptoms.

Hospice treats the whole patient, physically, emotionally and spiritually with understanding and support.

PROCEED WITH CAUTION

WHEN DO YOU CALL HOSPICE? EARLY AS POSSIBLE! Call hospice when you know there is no more treatment available. You will realize after reading this book that hospice could be years of living. So often our medical community squeezes your pocketbook as they offer hope for a cure. They leave you with the uncomfortable side effects and despair when they could have recommended hospice. Over and over I have witnessed a patient die on admission instead of living quality months on hospice. Remember, it is FREE if you are on Medicare. Ask your doctor to tell you when you have six months or less to live. Tell him to

"BE HONEST!"

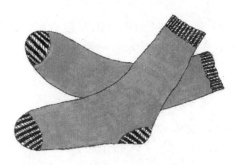

RED AND GREEN KNITTED SLIPPERS

Cold to the bone, I was searching for a patient's home interested in hospice on a snowy morning. The winding road was steep and the tires were slipping on icy black top. The car lacked chains. To be safe, I backed off the accelerator and put the transmission in first gear. The snow was quickly turning my red Mustang white as I searched for the address on frozen mail boxes.

Barely legible was "441" in black numbers on a mail box nailed to a leaning two by four. I slowly maneuvered my Mustang into the driveway and stopped behind an old black Ford pickup. Through my windshield I could see a small house nestled between two tall snow covered pine trees.

As I opened the car door the smell of burning wood drifted from the red painted brick chimney of the house. I was hoping the fire was keeping everyone warm, especially my prospective patient. My shoes made crunching sounds in the frozen snow as I walked around the truck. I knocked on the door, took an icy deep breath, and hoped for the best.

Every house is like a box of chocolates. You never know what you will find behind the front door.

A big burly man, with a red and black plaid flannel shirt, cracked open the door, exposed me to a big black barking dog. I strained to see if the dog was on a leash.

"Get back Killer. Get back." The plaid shirted man was trying to shove the dog back with his leg. The dog was not on a leash!

This dog does not like visitors!

I stepped back and waited.

A weak voice came from under a mound of covers on a bed across the room. I heard the snap of fingers. "Killer, come!" The barking stopped. The dog turned, walked across the room, and sat in front of the bed. A hand came slowly out from under the covers and took hold of the dog's collar

Somewhat relieved, I moved back to the threshold. "Hi, my name is Karen. I'm a hospice nurse looking for Joe Smith. Am I at the right house? Is Joe living here?"

"What's left of him," the burly man replied. "He's over there on the bed behind Killer. I'm his big brother. Can I take your bag?"

"Sure, it's heavy."

"Come on in and shut the door. You're heating up the outside."

"That's quite a purse you're draggin'."

"It's not my purse. It's my nursing bag. Thanks for your help."

"Wow, are you carrying a bowling ball in here? It sure feels like it!"

"No, it's the local hospice library, my phone, a few bandages, scissors, stethoscope, blood pressure cuff, and a scale!"

Standing in the middle of a worn wood floor, I looked across the room at Joe. Behind his bed was a big front window covered by old sheer curtains and shades half drawn. Dust and dirt covered the bare floor.

Joe's seventy-two years old and has advanced lung cancer metastasized to his bone.

Joe slowly pulled the covers from his head and smiled a toothless grin. He reached across with his empty hand to a small end table in front of a wall poster of Kobe Bryant dunking a basketball. He picked up his false teeth and slipped them into his mouth

Pretty adaptable for a man in bed on continuous oxygen. I hope he keeps holding on to that dog.

"I need my choppers if I'm gonna' talk." We all laughed out loud.

He looks like a permanent fixture in his bed.

Two women were sitting with their heads down on an old leather couch. They were knitting red and green slippers.

I'm not sure these ladies even know I'm here.

My doorman, who was still standing holding my black leather nursing bag, was motioning me towards the coffee pot brewing on the wood stove.

"Do you need a cup of hot coffee to warm you up?"

"Sounds great! It's cold out there and a cup of coffee will warm my cold hands and keep me going. Let me have my nursing bag."

Reaching for my nursing bag, I took a step towards Joe. Killer started growling, tugging at his collar, and showing his big yellow teeth. I saw the hair along his back stand on edge.

Backing behind a big worn chair full of clean linens and towels, I pointed at the dog. "That dog is too dangerous! If you don't restrain him, this visit will be over."

"Roger, put a leash on this dog and take him to the bedroom!"

Can Roger control Killer? I've had one dog bite already. Two's not a charm!

Roger took a leash hanging from a nail on the kitchen wall and hooked it to Killer's collar. Joe released Killer. As Roger dragged him across the floor, Killer attempted to lunge at me teeth bared. Roger restrained him with the leash and shoved him through the bedroom door. "I'll be happy when I don't have to deal with that damn dog!"

Joe motioned for me to come out from behind the chair. "Sorry about the dog. We'll keep him in the bedroom next time you come."

Where's a clean place to put my nursing bag. Can't set it on the floor. How about the chair with clean linens and towels?

The doorman handed me a cup of coffee. "Do you want sugar and cream?"

"No, I like it black. Thanks."

"Can I get you a chair?"

"Yes, please."

He found an old wooden folding chair leaning against the wall. He set it between the worn chair and Joe's bed.

"I'm Roger and these ladies are our wives, Leila and Lucy." Pointing to Joe, "He's the one you're here for."

Holding the hot cup of coffee between my hands, I sat in the creaky chair and turned my attention to Joe under a mountain of old blankets. He had a cute grin with his shining dentures.

"Joe, I'm here to talk to you about hospice."

Is Joe safe in this cluttered place? I'm not sure I'm safe on this chair!

"Hey Lucy, this woman here is gonna' talk about that hospice thing, you know. Help you while you're dyin' stuff."

One of the ladies lifted her head. "Sounds good to me." She went back to knitting.

He has less than six months to live.

"It's not about dying. It's about living as long as you can and being comfortable while you're alive."

"This isn't living, but I'm trying to hang on 'til Christmas."

He looked over at the ladies. "Did you hear that Lucy. At least I'd like to have one more Christmas with you."

One of the women nodded her head.

He has stage four cancer.

"I hope hospice can help you reach your goal. Christmas is a special day."

Propped up in the corner by the fireplace was an artificial Christmas tree. Only a broken angel hung from the top branch.

Will they decorate the tree before Christmas?

"Hospice can help you live here at home. Would you like that?"

"This ain't my home. I've been living here with my dog and wife at Roger's for over a year and I've been laying in this damn bed for the last three months. It wasn't my idea, but the economy's not like it used to be."

Joe scratched his bald head. "I would like to die somewhere else, but this is better than the hospital or an old folks home."

If Joe agrees, his end of life care will take place in Roger's home. His brother will be his primary caregiver.

"Did my doctor ask you to come?"

"Yes, I've spoken with her."

Joe tried to push himself up with his elbows onto his pillows. His purple tee shirt was emerging from under the covers showing part of a yellow sun.

"Your doctor asked if I would explain the hospice benefit. She feels hospice will help your family manage your care at home."

I took a sip of the strong coffee.

"After I tell you about hospice, you can decide to continue your ER visits or have me to help you here at home."

I took a gulp.

"If you choose hospice, you will not return to the oncology center for further treatments or to the ER for any life saving measures."

"You mean, if someone thinks I'm dying, I don't have to go to the hospital?"

5

"That's right! You won't be going to the hospital again." I took another sip, it was still hot. "Hospice is end of life care. It means you understand the doctor's diagnosis that you are nearing the end of life and you will die at home with your family, if possible. That day will come."

Joe looked at his wife who was counting her stitches. "Lucy, did you hear that? You can't keep me alive forever."

"Well, it's not like I haven't tried. You've been bouncing back and forth with those cancer treatments and radiation. You're like a living yoyo."

"Well, I think I'm ready to admit defeat, there is nothing more they can do with me."

Radiation and chemo, looks like it didn't help!

Joe pushed himself up a little further and the rising sun became a basketball with a 'Go Lakers' logo in black letters.

"Looks like you're a Lakers' fan. Roger, are you a Lakers' fan too?"

Roger pointed to the poster. "We're all ballers in this family. Right, Joe?"

Holding the cup in both hands, I drank a little more.

"Yep. I was a basketball player in high school but I started smokin' about fifty years ago. That ended my game! Smokin' finally caught up with me."

Joe reached for his oxygen tank and turned it off.

"It seemed at first I started coughin' in the mornings. I thought it was an allergy or a cold that wouldn't go away. Then I got short of breath. When I started coughin' up blood, Lucy had me go to the doctor."

He reached over to the table for a pack of cigarettes, tapped the pack on his palm. He took out a cigarette, and grabbed the lighter.

"That's when I found out I had lung cancer. Three rounds of chemo and radiation, but it didn't help, it made me sicker."

He pointed to the end table with a shoe box filled with prescription bottles. "Look at all those pills. You'd think I

6

was the pharmacy. All those pills haven't done one damn thing for me, except make me weaker. I know it's no use. Now I have to think about dyin'."

He placed the cigarette in his mouth.

He's not going to smoke, is he? Thank God he turned his O2 off.

Joe flicked his lighter, and took a puff.

"My bucket list is real short. I want to die without pain, if that's possible."

He waved his cigarette at the ladies. "I want someone to take care of my wife and Killer."

"Joe, I'm not a smoker. I'd appreciate it if you would put your cigarette out and wait until I leave before you light up again."

"Sorry." Joe quenched his cigarette into a filled ash tray beside his bed.

Brushing the smoke away, "I'll try to help you with your pain. Our social worker will help with your wife and Killer."

"Then I'm interested."

"You told me you are a basketball fan. I love your Lakers shirt and Kobe poster."

"Yeh. We all watch 'em when we can. Right Roger?"

"Yeh, I like Kobe, he's a good three point shooter. Best in the NBA!"

"Hospice is like a basketball team. When you have a basketball team you need a coach and an assistant coach, right? Your doctor is the head coach and our hospice doctor will be his assistant on call twenty-four hours a day."

Extending all five fingers, I held up my hand. I touched my thumb. "Joe, there's only one center and it'll be me, your nurse. When I'm off duty or sick, there will always be another nurse available for you, twenty-four hours a day, seven days a week."

Roger took a step towards us and took a sip of coffee as he watched me put up my first two fingers. "There will be

7

two forwards. One is the hospice volunteer who never gets a paycheck. The volunteer could be your friend and drop in whenever you need a helping hand. He's someone to keep you company or watch you while your family takes a break. The other forward will be a hospice chaplain who knows how to pray for you and offers spiritual support for you and your family."

Roger put his hand on the back of the worn chair, as I folded my first two fingers under my thumb and opened my ring and little fingers. "Joe, There'll be two guards on the team. First, there's the home health aide, who specializes in bubbles for your bath and other hygiene care. The second is the point guard, who's the hospice medical social worker. The social worker will make at least one mandatory visit to your home every month."

His brother leaned over the chair and piped up with a deep voice, "How much will hospice cost?"

"Nothing! There's never a bill. It's a benefit of Joe's Medicare"

"Do I need any other insurance?" Joe asked.

"No other insurance is needed unless you fall out of bed and break your leg. Hospice does not pay for that."

Roger moved all the linens and my nursing bag off the worn chair to the couch beside the girls. He sat down in the worn chair with his cup of coffee. "What about Joe's medications. Does he have a copay?"

"No copay! Hospice will keep you supplied with medications by reordering them through a local pharmacy. I'll check your meds when I see you every week. If you need a refill, I'll order them and have them delivered to your door."

"There's no charge for medications or medical equipment if it's for his comfort or related to his lung cancer. If there's a need for additional medications, I'll call your doctor for orders."

Lucy stopped knitting for a moment. "Who do we call in an emergency?"

"Glad you asked. Call the hospice number for any problems or emergencies, day or night. You will no longer be calling nine-one-one or going to the hospital unless I arrange it. I'll be your 'nurse angel,' always watching out for you and will call your doctor with updates in your care."

Joe pointed at me. "Stand up and turn around!"

"What for?"

"Just do it."

Standing up, I turned around reluctantly.

Did I spill coffee on my lab coat?

"I'm looking for your wings. Can't see your wings, but you have one helluva smile." I laughed.

Joe seems alert with his great sense of humor. I'll ask the basic questions.

"Joe, let me ask a few questions."

"Sure, shoot."

"What's your name?"

"Joe Smith."

"Where are you?"

"I'm where you are. Don't you know where you are?" I chuckled.

"I mean, what city?"

"Red Deer."

"What year is it?"

"Two thousand six?"

"Who's President?"

"Bill Clinton!" With a wink, "Don't we wish?"

Joe's not confused. He's able to make normal decisions, a necessary requirement to sign the consents.

"Joe, you're eligible for hospice. Do you want to give it a try?"

"Yep, I'm ready for the slam dunk! I want you for my cheerleader!"

9

"Roger, could you grab the clipboard in the outside pocket of my nursing bag? It has a hospice folder clipped to it."

Roger reached over to the couch, retrieved the clipboard, and gave it to me. I read and explained each consent in the folder. Joe signed it. I tore off the last sheet and placed it in his home folder. After the last consent, I slid the folder under the shoe box on the table.

The front copies of the consent forms went back into my nursing bag. After taking out my physical assessment sheet, I reached for my stethoscope and started Joe's physical. I listened to his heart and lung sounds, checked his blood pressure, and examined his skin from his head to toe, looking for pressure sores and abnormalities. I jotted this info on the assessment sheet.

He seems bed bound. I hope he doesn't try to navigate through this obstacle course! His legs are like toothpicks.

He had pressure sores on both ankle bones, tailbone, and on the soles of both feet.

Joe's been in bed three months? He hasn't been turning enough. He probably can't get out of bed.

Joe was lying in a make shift hospital bed, too short for him. His feet were pressing against a plywood board.

"Where did you get this bed?"

"My neighbor had this hospital bed. His wife died in it. He had it in his garage for scrap. He's loanin' it to me. It ain't got anyway to raise it, if that's what your lookin' for!"

I'll need to order him a longer hospital bed.

"Joe, can you get out of bed by yourself?"

"Hell no! That's why Roger's here!"

"He can only stand if I help him," Roger said as he sipped another swig of his cold coffee. "I can help him to his arm chair and to his commode thing when necessary, but it's killing my back."

He's bed bound. Does he need a Hoyer lift to protect Roger's back?

10

"Let me show you how to turn Joe safely in bed with a draw sheet. I completed my notes on the assessment sheet, placed it into my nursing bag.

"We start with bed in the flat position."

This bed doesn't move! It's always flat."

After standing up, I took a crumpled sheet from the end of the bed. "I want to teach you how to make a draw sheet in order to reposition Joe to the top of the bed."

"Fold the length in half and fold the width in half." I folded the sheet into a big rectangle.

"Roll half the rectangle to the middle." I rolled up half the rectangle.

"Roger, walk over to the other side of the bed." Roger laid his empty coffee cup on the floor and stood up.

He walked around to the other side of the bed.

"I'm bending his leg farthest from you. His foot is flat on the bed and the knee is bent. Now put you hand on that knee, other hand on his shoulder, pull both knee and leg towards you." Roger rolled Joe onto his side.

"Joe, how does it feel to be a human pretzel?"

"Not bad since you're here."

Leaning over I placed the rolled edge of the rectangle to his back. "You place the rolled portion of the draw sheet next to his lower back and hips."

"Before you turn him over the hump, you can give him a back rub. Roger, come over to this side and watch as I rub his back."

Grudgingly he walked to my side of the bed.

Seeing no lotion on the table, I walked to the couch and reached in my nursing bag for my Aveeno. "Watch and learn, Roger!" Returning and leaning towards Joe, I rubbed my lotioned hands up and down his bony back. He moaned in delight as I spread the lotion and kneaded it into his skin.

"You can do that all day."

"Not until I get my turn," Roger interjected.

11

"Roger, watch me as I roll Joe over the rolled up edge of the draw sheet." I reached for Joe's shoulder and gently pulled his back onto the bed over the hump. One by one I pulled his knees to an upright position. I extended his closest leg to me. "Roger now you pull on this bent knee and his far shoulder and gently roll them towards you until he's over the hump."

Now Joe was facing me on his side. I leaned over him and finished rubbing his back.

"Now go to the other side and unroll the draw sheet." Roger walked around to the other side of the bed and unrolled the draw sheet.

"Roll Joe onto his back." Roger pulled on his shoulder until he was on his back. Joe straightened his legs."

"Joe, are you still able to bend your knees?"

He nodded and winked.

"Now that you are flat on the bed we're going to give you a ride to the top. Bend your knees and dig your heels in. Are you ready?"

Joe bent his knees. "I'm ready!"

"Roger, take hold of the draw sheet with me. On the count of three we'll lift and Joe will push with his legs. This'll move him to the top." Roger took hold of the draw sheet with both hands.

"One, two, three ..." We slid Joe to the top of the bed. His feet stopped pressing against the plywood board. I placed a pillow between his feet and the board.

Roger smacked his hands together and looked at me. "We did it, job well done!" He turned to Joe. "Vaseline on your butt would make it a whole lot easier!"

"Roger, now you can teach Leila how to help position Joe."

"Watch as I place the pillows between his knees and heels. Do this every two or three hours. "This will prevent further pressure sores."

"He will have an alternating air pressure mattress which will prevent bed sores." I measured and cleansed all nine of his sores.

He has stage two and three decubitus. No wonder he's in pain.

I applied a Tegaderm on each wound and wrote the date on the dressing.

That gives him an extra layer of skin.

"Joe, are you in pain?"

"Hell yes, all the time."

"Where's your pain?" Point to it."

"All over!"

"What are you taking for pain?"

"Two horse pills."

I bet he's on plain Vicodin. He needs extra strength and closer intervals. Hope that'll be enough to stop his pain.

"On a scale of one to ten, if ten was the worst possible pain, what's your level of pain?"

"I don't know by numbers, but it's bad."

"I need to know. So try to think about your pain level by numbers. Zero is no pain, ten is screaming pain."

"It's maybe an eight or nine."

"I'll call your doctor and get a medication order for your pain. Let me get my cell phone."

After retrieving my cell phone from my nursing bag, I called his doctor and received an order to increase the dosage and change the interval to every three hours while awake and as necessary through the night.

I'll start a bowel regime of laxatives to help have bowel movements every day. Increase narcotics equals increased laxatives.

"Joe, you need to do some exercises to increase circulation to your legs and feet. Whenever you see a TV commercial wiggle your toes, move your feet in circles, and bend your knees." I lifted the covers to watch him circle his feet.

13

"Roger, I'm going to leave a fractured bedpan (smaller in height bedpan) in case you can't get him to his commode. This will keep from putting extra pressure on his tailbone sore when he's having a bowel movement."

"Excuse me for a few minutes. I have to go out to my car and get your bedpan." I brushed the snow off the trunk, searched for the key hole, chipped off the ice, and opened the lid to my hospice central supply room.

Wow, a frozen bed pan. This will wake everything up!

When I returned holding his pink bedpan and milk colored urinal, Joe smiled, reached under the covers, pulled out a Folger's coffee can, and held it up so everyone could see. "Look here, Lucy. I can get rid of my old piss can. Now I have a plastic milk bottle shaped like a duck!" We all laughed hysterically.

"Soon you'll have an extra-long hospital bed with a remote control. You'll have fun with your built in roller coaster."

"Roger, do you have queen size sheets?"

"Yes, that's the size of our bed. I guess I can share a sheet with you, Joe."

"Roger, I don't want you to hurt your back so I'll order a mechanical lift to get Joe in and out of bed safely. I'll schedule a visit when the equipment company arrives to show you how to use the Hoyer lift. It will prevent Joe from falling and save your back."

Roger's back is very important now.

Joe propped himself up on his elbows. "I don't need your damn lift! Can't you see we have enough in this house? It's already a hospital!"

Roger put his hand on Joe's shoulder. "Come on Joe. I think that will help me a lot. You know, I'm not as young as I used to be."

"It's portable," I added. "Put it wherever you have room. Use it when you need it. Joe, it'll help you get out of bed to your commode and allow you to sit in a chair."

"Well, okay. If it'll help Roger, I can give it a try."

There was a choice of two nursing visits a week. Joe chose one. He agreed to meet with the social worker.

"How about that volunteer?" Roger asked. "Leila and I are members of a bowling team. The league plays every Thursday morning at ten. Lucy'd like to bowl, but she has to stay home with Joe. A volunteer would let Lucy join us."

"I'll talk with our volunteer coordinator and see if she can find a volunteer awake at nine in the morning."

"Joe, would you like a chaplain visit?"

"Hell, no! After what I saw in Viet Nam, I never believed there was a God. If there is a God, why wouldn't he have stopped those commies in Viet Nam or those Germans who caused the Holocaust? No way! Count me out."

"I'll assign you a home health aide twice a week for your bed baths. How does that sound?"

Lucy was exuberant. "Oh goodie! He needs a bath every day. He might even enjoy it!"

Joe gave her 'the look.' "You had better behave yourself and be here to supervise!"

He needs a fun loving aid to roll with the punches. Not everyone can handle this vet.

"Where is the folder I brought with me? It's bright orange."

"It's here on the table." Roger retrieved the bright orange home folder from under the shoe box and handed it to me. "In this folder is an important blue paperback pamphlet called *Gone from My Sight*. Please take time to read it. It's full of information about dying at home. If you have any questions, write them down so we can discuss them at our next visit."

Leila stopped knitting. "Will there be a test?"

"No, ... well, maybe." I winked at her, reached in my nursing bag for a hospice magnet, placed it on their metal file cabinet, and put stickers on their phones with our hospice phone number.

"Be sure to call if Joe's still in pain after taking his new medication." I hugged Joe and each family member.

Joe lifted his skinny arm and gave me the peace sign. "Thanks. Don't fall in the ditch on your way out the driveway."

"I'll try not to."

Could happen with all the snow!

I heard Killer barking and scratching at the door.

Can I slip him a dog treat?

I stopped, pulled out a zip lock bag of doggy treats from my bag. "Can I give Killer a small doggy bone under the door?"

"Sure, why not? Maybe that will shut him up."

"Here's your treat, Killer. I'll be back. Take good care of Joe." His growling stopped for a moment.

Maybe he'll remember me.

"Good bye Joe. I'll see you in two days. Call me if you need anything."

After returning to the office, I talked to the hospice volunteer director. I was delighted when she found a match for Joe, another Viet Nam vet.

On my visits I always greeted him the same way. "Hello, handsome."

Joe would tease me. "Where're your glasses?"

I don't even own a pair, yet!

He was full of jokes, always trying to make me laugh.

He shared some horrifying memories while fighting in Vietnam. He told me how lucky he was to survive the war as a Marine and to live another fifty years.

"Karen, I think I'm ready for the hereafter."

Thinking he might be ready for a chaplain visit, I asked, "What's the 'hereafter?'"

"It's what comes after here," he whispered. "Plain nothin'!"

"To me it's heaven."

"It's not heaven to me. When you're dead, you're dead, like a dog."

Each time I made a visit, Lucy was sitting in the same spot on the old worn out couch. I would sit with her after I took care of Joe. She loved to reminisce her memories of living with Joe in Arkansas.

In one of those conversations, Lucy mentioned two big problems. "Karen, where am I going to live after my husband dies? ... And what about Killer? I don't think Roger and Leila want him or me. By then we will have outlived our welcome."

"Lucy, these are big concerns. I'll refer them to our social worker. She'll call you tomorrow and schedule a visit." I reached out and gave her a hug. "We'll find a place for you."

The social worker helped the family make plans for Lucy to live with her daughter. The daughter worked part time, lived on a horse ranch out of state, and had plenty of room for Killer and Lucy.

As the Christmas holidays approached, he was taking stronger pain medications and seemed comfortable. Joe was still hoping his body would last until Christmas.

Roger's wife decorated the green artificial tree with red knitted ornaments and little white twinkling lights. She was trying to keep Joe's spirit alive. Joe was fading, like a flower fades under the heat of the desert sun.

A week before Christmas, Lucy asked me, "Is red your favorite color?"

"Why would you think that?"

"You drive a red Mustang."

"You're right. Red is my favorite color. My car is red. My front door is red. My dog has a red collar. I was born in Nebraska and we all know the 'Big Red' college football team is number one."

Lucy smiled and nodded. "Red is the color of Christmas too. It's almost here and I think Joe's going to make it."

I doubt it if he'll make it. Cancer is winning this fight.

"But he doesn't talk to me anymore and only drinks a little orange juice each morning with his medicine. He refuses to get out of bed and keeps pointing at Killer. I think his memory is leaving him. I keep reminding him Killer will go with me to our daughter's house. I don't think he remembers."

His appetite is gone. I hope he can make it to Christmas for her sake.

On Christmas Eve day I dropped in and found Joe sleeping. Killer woke him up with his barking.

"Merry Christmas, Joe." I kissed him on the forehead and held his hand. "Joe, are you comfortable? Squeeze my hand if you're in pain."

He did not respond. "Roger, when was the last time you gave him his pain medication?"

"I gave him 'Roxy' about four hours ago. He seems to be comfortable. He's sleeping most of the time anyway."

It was time for another dose of Roxanol. "Roger, give him Roxanol every two hours to keep ahead of his pain. If he awakens in the night, give him an additional dose. Remember if there is no relief, call us for further orders."

Reaching in my hospice bag, I took out a Christmas gift bag of my favorite homemade sugar cookies shaped like angels, handed it to Lucy, and wished them a Merry Christmas.

On my phone call with Lucy on Christmas day, she told me Joe was still alive and seemed comfortable. He spent the day sleeping. "We put a Santa hat on Joe while Roger walked around with his Rudolf antlers. Santa brought Joe a large red flannel shirt to lay over him, like another blanket, to keep him cozy."

He must have smelled the turkey with all the trimmings.

I got a call two days after Christmas. Joe had stopped breathing. "Would you come right away to be with Lucy?"

When I arrived she was sobbing with tears of grief mingled with tears of relief while still holding Joe's cold hand. I hugged her and simply said, "He's out of pain, no longer a prisoner in a body too weak to hold him."

Lucy looked into my teary green eyes. "Look, he has two pairs of my knitted slippers on his feet. At least his feet are warm."

I checked his feet and found both red and green slippers on each foot. I smiled.

With the help of the family, I called the necessary phone numbers.

Lucy called her daughter. "Dad is gone." She broke down in tears. "Can you come see me? I'm ready to be with you." She continued the conversation, then hung up the phone. "Karen, it would have been nice if we could have been with her. But she couldn't live with Joe's anger and harsh words."

We moved to the table in the kitchen. Lucy and I drank hot peppermint tea while Roger and his wife chose mugs of strong black coffee. I listened to many wonderful memories of Joe.

He was quite a character.

The mortuary assistants arrived to take his body. Lucy kissed him on the forehead to say good-by. She asked that they keep his head uncovered as he went out the door. Roger and his wife gently patted him on his shoulder. It was the last time they would see him. He had told them to cremate his body. Roger and Killer, on his leash, followed Joe to the front door. Killer walked with his tail and head down.

It seems he knows Joe is gone.

We returned to the table where Roger ended our sharing time. "We all knew he was leaving us when he could no longer eat, drink, or holler at the dog." He stood up and raised his red Christmas mug and made a toast. "Here's to

19

my brother Joe. He liked the year two thousand six and wanted to end the year wearing Lucy's red and green hand knitted slippers. Good choice, Joe. Stay warm my friend. We'll miss you."

We clinked our cups together and drank.

Lucy got up from the round table and walked over to the Christmas tree's blinking lights. She reached under the branches for a little red package tied with a big white bow. She returned, gave me a hug, kissed my cheek, and handed me the present. "Open it. It's for you."

I slowly opened it, saving the ribbon and paper. Much to my surprise, in it was a pair of beautiful soft cuddly red Angora slippers!

She wanted me to try them on. When I modeled them, they were a perfect fit! She insisted I wear them home to keep my feet warm inside my cowboy boots.

Roger gave me a 'wolf whistle.' "You're the first angel with red slippers I've ever seen.

As I promised Joe, there was no sheriff, no coroner, no autopsy, and no EMT to resuscitate him.

This is dignity in dying.

I'm happy Joe chose hospice. If the family had not chosen hospice, they would be seeing a coroner, a sheriff, an ambulance, and an EMT team starting CPR and an IV to revive him. Probably, even a little rib cracking...

Roger was the primary caregiver but Leila and Lucy assisted him. Through good times and bad, they provided care for Joe, every hour of the day.

It's unusual for a family to work together to avoid hiring a caregiver. They chose to be Joe's caregiver, a most difficult task, and equally shared the load. They're my 'A Team.' I'm sure it changed the way they look at the gift of life.

I'll wear my red knitted slippers Lucy gave me to remind me of Joe and his family, especially on Christmas Eve.

As I was leaving, Lucy followed me out to my car. "Karen, I know Joe didn't believe in the hereafter. He thought death was the end. I think when he died, something left him. I think angels came last night and took him somewhere."

Those angels are dancing and wearing their red and green knitted slippers, hand knitted by Lucy.

DEATH IS NOTHING AT ALL
Canon Henry Scott-Holland
Canon of St Paul's Cathedral
1847-1918

Death is nothing at all.
It does not count.
I have only slipped away into the next room.
Nothing has happened.
Everything remains exactly as it was.
I am I, and you are you, and the old life that we lived so
     fondly together is untouched, unchanged.
Whatever we were to each other, that we are still.
Call me by the old familiar name.
Speak of me in the easy way which you always used.
Put no difference into your tone.
Wear no forced air of solemnity or sorrow.
Laugh as we always laughed at the little jokes that we
     enjoyed together.
Play, smile; think of me; pray for me.
Let my name be ever the household word that it always was.
Let it be spoken without an effort, without the ghost of a
     shadow upon it.
Life means all that it ever meant.
It is the same as it ever was.
There is absolute and unbroken continuity.
What is this death but a negligible accident?
Why should I be out of mind because I am out of sight?

21

I am but waiting for you, for an interval, somewhere very
    near, just round the corner.
All is well.
Nothing is hurt; nothing is lost.
One brief moment and all will be as it was before.
How we shall laugh at the trouble of parting when we meet
    again!

From: 'The King of Terrors,' a sermon on death delivered in
    St Paul's Cathedral on Whitsunday 1910, while the
    body of King Edward VII was lying in state at
    Westminster: Published in *Facts of the Faith, 1919*

PARTING

Bruce Farr
2014

Come love, walk with me,

Hold my hand along the restless sea.

Tomorrow my touch may be no more,

Pausing, to meet on another shore.

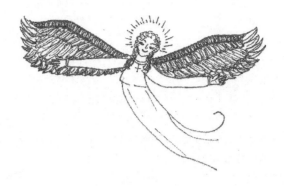

HEAVEN ... I'VE BEEN THERE!

Upon arrival at the Foothill Apartments, the elevator was in sight, but the staircase was closer. My body needed the exercise so I climbed the endless staircase.

This will be my cardio for the day.

At the second floor I paused to rest.

"Hu, hu, hu ...," I was breathing deeply.

Should have taken the elevator!

I laughed at myself.

I guess my marathon days are over!

Going down the hallway looking for room 311, I began humming the 'old spiritual.' "I am climbing Jacob's ladder,"

When I reached her door, I took a deeper breath, and looked at my watch.

Good. I'm on time. ... No doorbell? Oh well...

My humming changed to singing as I swung my nursing bag over my shoulder, and began knocking on the door in rhythm.

Life would be much easier if every house had a doorbell!

No response! I hollered, "Hello! Is anyone home?"

"I hear you. Give me a minute. I'm coming." The door swung open. A woman stood peering over her glasses, staring at my lab coat. She was trying to read my name badge.

It's even difficult for me to read. I wish they'd use bigger letters.

"You must be the nurse we're expecting." It was a matter of fact tone of voice.

"You're right. I'm Karen. I'm looking for Judith. What's your name?"

"I'm her daughter, Melinda. Come in." She pointed to a chubby woman on a gold plaid couch as she limped to a Lazy Boy chair. "This is my mother, Judith."

"Hi Judith ..."

She interrupted, "Don't forget to introduce Marianne, our calico cat, who sits on the window sill. She thinks she's a watch cat. She was meowing before you started knocking on the door."

Pointing to Melinda's knee, "My daughter had knee surgery two weeks ago. It takes her a while to get up. Sorry for the delay. Come sit on the couch with me."

After placing my nursing bag at the end of the couch, I sat beside her.

Judith started the conversation as the cat hid behind the couch. "I heard you singing outside my door. Will you be my singing nurse?"

She's alert and oriented.

"Yes, I will. I love to sing."

Judith is seventy years old with end stage chronic obstructive pulmonary disease (COPD).

"Lucky for you! I love to sing too, but I'm out of breath most of the time."

Her fingertips and lips have a slightly purplish blue color.

"How much oxygen are you using?"

Her oxygen comes from a portable tank.

24

"I keep it at two liters."

Her breathing is semi-rapid and shallow.

"How long has it been at two liters?"

"Months! It's good for talking, but not for singing."

"Are you aware of what Hospice is?"

"No, only what I've heard from my neighbor. She says it's about dying at home."

"No, it's about living each day with comfort and dignity, preparing you and your family for your last day. It's one of the best kept secrets in America. Our hospice team will support you every day, right here in your home."

Judith nodded her head. "Oh, you can arrange help for me at home? I really want to be home when I die."

"Hospice will not pay the rent or stay with you twenty four hours a day. It will put in place a team of professionals to assist you in your needs, and be available for any concerns or emergencies twenty-four hours a day, seven days a week."

"Hospice is like a wheel." Pointing to the palm of my hand, "The hub of the wheel is you, the patient, and your family. Everyone on the team will listen to your concerns and wishes."

Holding up my index finger, "I am the first spoke of the wheel, the hospice case manager, a registered nurse. I am responsible for communicating with all the other members of the hospice team."

Adding my middle finger, "The second spoke is the home health aide who is responsible for your hygiene."

Touching my ring finger, "The third spoke is the medical social worker who listens to your concerns and offers community resources and emotional support."

Holding up four fingers, "The fourth spoke will be the chaplain, who offers spiritual counsel for you and your family."

Showing her all my fingers, "The fifth spoke is a volunteer. This trained volunteer becomes a good friend to help you and your family."

Circling my hand, "The rim is the doctors."

"Who's going to order my medicine if I have more than one doctor?"

"Your primary care doctor."

"What if you can't get a hold of him? You know I sometimes can't reach him."

"We have a doctor on call. She's our hospice director. If we can't reach your doctor, she'll order your medications."

"What's her name?"

"Her name is Dr. Singh. If you need her, she can come to your home."

Judith pointed around the room with her open hand. "Karen, this really isn't my home. This is my son's apartment. I had to sell my condo. I needed the money for my medical bills."

"I'm sorry to hear that."

"Here's good news. You will never get a hospice bill. You may still have to make a few co-pays for meds not related to your hospice diagnosis."

My hand reached for the consents in my nursing bag. "One of the requirements is you must have a primary caregiver. Is your son going to be available?"

"I think so. I've been living with him for the last two years. He works during the day and is home during the night. He knows I will come back and haunt him, if he makes me die in an old-folks home or alone in some hospital!"

She looked at me square in my green eyes and remarked, "If I had wanted to die in a hospital, I wouldn't have asked Dr. Whittaker about hospice!"

My eyes glanced at the first consent form. "Here's a question I'm required to ask. The hospice admissions form asks for your spiritual preference. Do you have one?"

"I'm not religious, but I do have a personal relationship with God. Before you arrived today, I prayed for guidance regarding hospice."

"Would you like to have a chaplain visit?"

Judith smiled. "Yes, I'd appreciate that. I hope he'll talk about heaven."

"I am sure he will."

She leaned towards me, squeezed my hand, and whispered, "Heaven, I've already been there! I know how beautiful and tranquil it is."

"Really? You've been there? Tell me more."

"I was a young mother at home when my appendix ruptured. Back then, there were no antibiotics available. They rushed me to the hospital with a fever of over one hundred four degrees. I went into septic shock and lost consciousness." Judith placed her hand on her chest. "My heart stopped and the doctors pronounced me dead."

Judith began to raise both hands palms up towards the ceiling. "I remember floating from my bed through a tunnel towards a brilliant light. The light was a brilliant radiating white, whiter than I'd ever seen. I saw beautiful vibrant colors, colors I've never seen here on earth. The music was harmonious and brilliant, similar, but richer than a symphony orchestra. I can't find words to describe it."

She folded her hands in her lap. "I was resting in tranquil peace. There was a feeling of love, a feeling of being at home, belongingness. It was God's peace enveloping me."

"A man appeared reaching his hand out to me. He was dressed in a white robe."

"He said, 'Welcome to heaven. Follow me.'"

"I took his hand and started to walk with him. Then I remembered my children. I asked myself, 'Who was going to care for them?'"

"I pleaded with him. 'Please, let me return to take care of my two children.'"

"He turned to me. 'You can go back to your children. Remember to raise them for me.'"

"The last thing I remembered was the smile on his face and the scars on his wrists." She opened her hands and looked at her wrists.

"I came unexpectedly back to life. The doctors were astounded."

"I was disappointed to leave that heavenly realm. But on the other hand, I was very happy he gave me another chance. It was bitter sweet."

Judith bent forward and put her hand on my knee. "This time when I die, I know I will be in heaven forever. I only tell you this experience so you can share with others. Tell them death is not painful, it's peaceful! I have no fear of death for I know it'll be far better there than it is here."

"This I know for sure, life is short, and eternity is sure."

I'm feeling goose bumps. Maybe they're God bumps. What a story! I can't imagine having an after death experience!

"Judith, do you understand that on hospice we don't perform any heroic efforts to keep you alive?"

"It's like I told you. I don't want any efforts to keep me alive. When I die, promise me, you won't bring me back. Please, let me go!"

"Judith, that's one of our rules. No one will do CPR or take other measures to bring you back. You will die with dignity."

"Karen, just call me Judy?"

"Okay, I'll call you Judy. Did I tell you about the medications?"

"You told me there would be no bills."

Her large blue pill box is open on the table and it looks full and running over.

"Hospice pays for all your medications related to your diagnosis of COPD and those for your comfort. I'll reorder your meds as needed at each visit and our pharmacy will deliver them to your door."

"In my wildest dreams, I never thought my medications would be coming to my front door. It sounds like hospice will not only help me, but be available to help my family. Now they won't have to go the pharmacy. It's more than I expected. It's free! Sign me up!"

"How are you feeling about this, Melinda?"

"I'm okay. I want what would be best for mom." She turned to Judy. "Mom, I don't want to lose you."

"It's not my decision. It's God's."

"Yes, that's true. Mom, I think hospice will help you and I'm sure we'll need all the help we can get." Melinda moved closer to her mom, put her loving arms around her, and began to cry. "I love you so much, mom. Do what you think is best."

I gave Melinda a tissue and continued through the tears. I explained each of the consent forms in my hand. Judy willingly signed them.

By this time Marianne was rubbing my leg. I reached down to pet her and she jumped into Judy's lap. "Call hospice for any accident in the home or problems, even if you get bit by your cat! Does Marianne bite?"

"She can if she's cornered and frightened."

I'll be careful not to frighten her!

"Judy, this is our last consent form. Rights and Responsibilities. We call it the R&R form."

I wish it meant rest and relaxation. Wouldn't it be nice?"

"Judy, here are your responsibilities. Be home whenever a visit is scheduled. Never call nine-one-one. Keep your home safe."

Judy signed it.

"You need to keep your house safe for you and your caregivers. When we finish the physical assessment, I'll look around to see if there are any safety suggestions."

Judy is a brittle diabetic requiring insulin twice a day.

Listening with my stethoscope to her lungs, I heard expiratory wheezing and fluid bilaterally.

She has rales in both lungs. She needs her oxygen.

"Hospice will pay for your oxygen and breathing treatment supplies. I'll order you an oxygen concentrator. You'll use the tanks only in an emergency, when the electricity is off."

Her vital signs were normal, weight was one hundred ninety, and skin was dry and intact.

"Would you like a hospital bed so you can keep your head elevated? That will make it easier to breathe at night."

"No, I like my own queen size bed. It has two wedge bolsters, five soft pillows, including a long pink body pillow, piled high on my memory foam mattress. I'm used to being propped up in bed."

"Judy, I love your red four by four with a seat. Use it every day. Your walker will prevent a fall."

After a quick walk through her son's apartment, I found no apparent safety problems.

Before leaving, I copied every prescription and supplement on her med profile. I placed her paper work in an orange hospice folder and left it on the coffee table.

"Each visiting member of our team will use this folder. They will date and sign the blue sheet."

"There's a list of all of your medications. I'll update it as they change. Your consents are here along with other information."

Taking out a blue pamphlet from the folder, I said, "Please take time to read this pamphlet *Gone from my Sight.*" I handed the folder and pamphlet to Judy.

"Melinda, you and Jeff should read it too."

She's a teacher. She'll read it. I'm not sure about Jeff!
Melinda walked me to the door.

I hope Judy tells me more about what she saw in heaven. Everyone wants to know if heaven is real. I'll take the elevator down.

On my Tuesday and Friday visits I poked Judy's finger for a random blood sugar level, reviewed her home folder, checked her blood pressure, and listened to her lungs. At the end of the visits I compared her medications with her med profile, packed her pill box, ordered her refills and breathing treatment meds, and called her doctor for orders.

Judy allowed the real 'angels of hospice' to come three times a week to assist her. They bathed her, trimmed her nails, and checked her skin. They were responsible to report any skin abnormalities and changes in her comfort level. During their hourly visit they listened to Judy's concerns and offered emotional support.

Hugs can break down any wall.

Judy strongly disliked her walker. "I hate this walker, especially for short distances. It bangs up Jeff's walls and he lets me know! This is my four-by-four out of control."

Each week she complained of being tired and unable to walk. I ordered a wheelchair and a long extension tube for her oxygen concentrator.

As the weeks passed she had increased shortness of breath and swelling of her ankles and feet. Her labile blood sugar levels required doctor orders for titrating her insulin dose.

She took sedatives for sleep.

Judy shared her concerns, especially about Jeff's money management. "Jeff comes home from his job exhausted every evening. He does the shopping and usually buys TV dinners for my meals. He always buys the wrong toilet paper. I like Charmin for my softer places, but he refuses to spend the extra money."

31

Each visit I kept in communication with Jeff by writing him notes. I would emphasize it was important to call hospice about any change in her condition. When I mentioned the toilet paper problem, like magic, soft pink toilet paper rolls appeared in her bathroom.

How true is the saying, the little things in life are really the big things.

Death was an open subject. Judy referred to her passing with the term "my D-day." She was confident, always looking with anticipation to the tranquil setting she had seen as a young mother.

During one of my regular visits, Judy shared a unique request. "Karen, I want to be baptized before I die. It must be immersion, not sprinkling."

Sprinkling would be simple to arrange, but immersion was a bit more complicated. I referred her request to our chaplain. Judy was challenging him to do what no other chaplain had done, baptize a wheelchair bound hospice patient.

The plan was to have the baptism in her nephew's swimming pool. The hospice team worked together with the chaplain to make it happen. Her friends, relatives, and the hospice team were present.

It was a warm summer Saturday. The chaplain and I were in bathing suits covered with long sleeved white shirts and slacks.

There were only three steps into the shallow end. Gripping the rail and my arm, Judy stepped slowly into the water.

When the water was above her waist the chaplain asked, "Judy, why are you being baptized?"

"The Bible says, 'Believe and be baptized.' I want to let everyone know I have accepted Jesus as my Savior. By being baptized, I am identifying myself with his death, burial, and resurrection. It won't get me to heaven. It is an outward sign of my inward faith."

She wants everyone to know of her decision to follow Jesus.

The chaplain looked down at Judy. "You are a courageous woman. I would like to pray for you. Let's bow our heads."

The chaplain gave a short prayer. "I now baptize you in name of the Father, the Son, and the Holy Spirit." He covered her face with a folded white linen handkerchief, lowered her backwards into the water, and completely immersed her. I saw joy radiating from her face as he lifted her out of the water.

Tears are rolling down my cheeks. I think only Judy and her angels can see them.

Judy and I changed our clothes and joined her guests. The family had a bar-b-que with potato salad, baked beans, a decorated cake, and cookies. One by one her friends and family offered their congratulations.

Cool thing, being baptized in a pool instead of a church! She's enjoyed the attention and love.

Judy's faithful daughter, who lived close by, called weekly for updates. During one of those calls I encouraged Melinda to think about a full time caregiver. "Your mother is having increased shortness of breath. She also has difficulty wheeling herself from room to room, putting her TV dinners in the microwave, and getting off the toilet. She will soon need a full time caregiver."

The time arrived when Judy fell. With the cell phone in her pocket, she called Jeff at work. He called hospice and they notified me.

Forget this lunch. How bad is she hurt?

On my cell phone I called Judy. "I'll be there in five minutes."

When I arrived Judy was still on the bathroom floor. I called the non-emergency number of the fire department. They sent out strong young men to help Judy back into her wheelchair.

Seeing these strong good looking firemen makes tax paying easy.

She had sprained her wrist and had several skin tears. I cleansed her wounds, covered them with Neosporin, and bandaged them with non-adhesive dressings and paper tape. I was fortunate to find a bag of frozen peas. I placed it on her swollen wrist. She could move it in full rotation without pain.

"Try to keep these peas or ice on your wrist for fifteen minutes and off for thirty, repeating this through the day, until I check on you tomorrow. Can you do that?"

"I'll do my best."

I'm thankful she didn't break her wrist. We need to keep her safe.

The fall prompted a family meeting with the social worker. We needed to discuss Judy's safety during the time she was home alone. She would soon be bed bound. Being bed bound would require a hospital bed, an air pressure mattress, and a full time caregiver.

At the family meeting, Melinda decided to go on personal leave from her teaching job. Melinda was part 'earth angel' to become a full time caregiver like her mother had been for her as a child.

Child/parent role reversal, usually what goes around comes around!

Judy never forgot I could sing. She frequently asked me to sing her favorite hymns. Her two favorite songs were *Swing Low Sweet Chariot* and *Amazing Grace*.

She longs for her chariot and her ride into glory.

She was never depressed or afraid to die. She would remind me of heaven, her final home. At every visit she reminded me of the tranquility and peace she experienced. It helped her through the long hours of waiting.

Judy did not require pain medication.

This is unusual.

She complained of being too weak to get out of bed. "It's time now to stay in bed and let your daughter help you."

Even with this change in activity, she complained of being very short of breath. I called her doctor. He increased her oxygen concentration and approved the use of an oxygen mask. He changed the dosage of Xanax to help her relax.

During the next three weeks, Melinda complained about her mother's lack of appetite. "Karen, I've been feeding mom a scrambled egg in the mornings. She used to eat all of it, but now she only picks at it. It's true with the rest of her meals. She doesn't eat enough to keep a bird alive. It frustrates me."

"''It's okay. Her body can't utilize the food. Her metabolism is slowing down. Soon she'll have no appetite and refuse to eat. Never force her to eat."

Her insulin injections and oral medications stopped when she refused to eat or drink.

This dying process will take Judy at least three days without fluids for her kidneys to stop functioning and all systems to close down, a domino effect. Death is more difficult than being born because it takes much longer. Both birth and death lead to new life.

Melinda was very loving and attentive during Judy's dying process as she gave the appropriate sub-lingual medications and breathing treatments. The medications helped Judy's body relax and breathe easier.

During the active dying process, I visited Judy daily. Each time I held her hand and sang old spiritual song.

It won't be long now until you see your King,
It won't be long now until you see your King,
It won't be long now until you see your King,
Praise the Lord, Praise the Lord, you're going to see your
    King.

She relaxed and smiled. She knew what it meant. She would give me a double 'thumbs up.'

On the following Sunday morning the answering service connected me to Melinda. She had an urgency in her voice. "Mom's breathing is different, even after her breathing treatment. She's gasping, like, she can't get enough air. Can you come and check on her?"

"Of course I'll come. Is her oxygen mask in place?"

"She's wearing her oxygen mask."

"How many liters is she using?"

"I think three."

"Raise it to four. When was the last time you gave her Roxanol?"

"I gave it three hours ago."

"Go ahead and repeat the dose of point seven-five milliliters under her tongue. It will help her relax and breathe easier. It sounds like her 'D-day' is finally here."

"I think so. She needs to hear you sing to her one more time before she leaves. Mom will know your voice. I need you too!"

As soon as I arrived, I began softly singing "We are Climbing Jacob's Ladder" with new words:

Judy's climbing God's big ladder,
Judy's climbing God's big ladder,
Judy's climbing God's big ladder,
Soldier of the cross.

Witnessing the exchanging of her first breath of life with her last breath, I watched as she gave it back to her God. Her death was peaceful. She left us with a smile on her face, holding the hands of her son and daughter. She returned to that tranquil land of heaven.

Here I am attending the death of another friend. I am again feeling the presence of angels. The scriptures tell me God assigns angels to guard us throughout our lives. Each

36

of us must have personal angels who are with us from the moment of birth until the moment of death. The same angels who guarded her through life were probably those who attended her at death.

Psalm 91:11 tells us about guardian angels. "He shall give His angels charge over you, to guard you in all your ways."

That is why I believe I am dancing among 'guardian angels.' It is a sacred moment. It is one I cherish.

I am dancing with angels and I feel their wings all around me at the time of death!

Judy left this earth at seventy. She fulfilled her promise to raise her children for God. She had experienced a changed heart, become a faithful mother, and lived long enough to tell her heaven story.

She saw heaven open before her eyes for the second time. For Judy it was an instant transformation, passing from temporal into eternal life.

Judy told me something I have never forgotten. "Eternity is only a breath away for all of us. You should live faithful to the Holy Word of God. You will be an example for your children and all those you meet in life."

For you were buried with Christ when you were baptized. And with him you were raised to a new life because you trusted the mighty power of God, who raised Christ from the dead. Colossians 2:12

For me to live is Christ and to die is gain.
Philippians 1:21

PREPARING A PLACE
John 14:1-4
Jesus

"Let not your hearts be troubled; you believe in God, believe also in me.

In my Father's house are many mansions; if it were not so, I would have told you. I go to prepare a place for you.

And if I go and prepare a place for you, I will come again and receive you unto myself, that where I am, you may be there also.

And where I go, you know, and the way you know.

Thomas said to him, "Lord, we don't know where you go; how can we know the way?"

Jesus said to him, "I am the way, the truth and the life. No man comes to the Father, but by me. If you have known me, you have known the Father also. From here on you know him, and have seen him." (NEV)

A MOTHER'S LOVE
Howard Ellowis

Thirty five years have gone by since my mother's passing.
Only during fleeting moments has the thought of her crossed
     my mind.
In the years that she lived I remember only tenderness,
     protectiveness, and loving care.

My father, a rageaholic, critical and physically abusive
     managed to stay in my mind.
To my shame I have remembered only the bad in my
     upbringing, not the good.
Hurt, pain and fear took precedence over a mother's love.
Now that this realization has come to me, I want to live my
     life differently.
I want only to remember the good and to forget the bad.
This I can do if I am given the gift of time and will.
In longing and prayer I ask for it.

(Used by permission of the author)

THROUGH DIM EYES
Ella Wheeler Wilcox

Is it the world, or my eyes, that are sadder?
I see not the grace that I used to see
In the meadow-brook whose song was so glad, or
In the boughs of the willow tree.
The brook runs slower--its song seems lower
And not the song that it sang of old;
And the tree I admired looks weary and tired
Of the changeless story of heat and cold.

When the sun goes up, and the stars go under,
In that supreme hour of the breaking day,
Is it my eyes, or the dawn, I wonder,
That finds less of the gold, and more of the gray
I see not the splendor, the tints so tender,
The rose-hued glory I used to see;
And I often borrow a vague half-sorrow
That another morning has dawned for me.

When the royal smile of that welcome comer
Beams on the meadow and burns in the sky,
Is it my eyes, or does the Summer
Bring less of bloom than in days gone by?
The beauty that thrilled me, the rapture that filled me,
To an overflowing of happy tears,
I pass unseeing, my sad eyes being
Dimmed by the shadow of vanished years.

When the heart grows weary, all things seem dreary;
When the burden grows heavy, the way seems long.
Thank God for sending kind death as an ending,
Like a grand Amen to a minor song.

(Public domain)

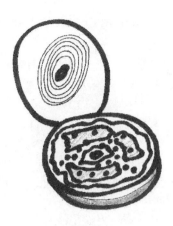

BAGELS AND LOX

The 'early bird gets the worm' took on a brand new meaning when I was asked to start my working day an hour earlier. The sun was about to rise when I found the big yellow house with a white porch encircling it.

Finding a yellow house with the right address is a big challenge at early dawn. It's always nice when the address is printed on the curb!

The big white front door had a sign fixed above the frame in bright capital red letters, 'WELCOME.'

Front doors intrigue me. Their handles and door knockers are as unique as the people who live inside.

On the right side of the door frame was a slanted ornate silver mezuzah.

This must be a Jewish family.

The door opened quickly after I pressed the brass doorbell. I was surprised to see a tall handsome muscular man with a trimmed black beard dressed in green scrubs.

"Hi, you must be the hospice nurse I'm expecting. You're here for my mother, Sara. I'm Dr. Weinstein, Sara's son. You can call me Dr. John. Come in."

"Yes, I'm the hospice nurse. Call me Karen."

"I have a hip replacement this morning. I don't have a lot of time."

Dr. John worked at the local regional hospital. He was an orthopedic surgeon.

Glancing around the living room I found my patient lying motionless in a hospital bed which I had ordered.

"Please come with me." Dr. John led me into his huge modern kitchen. "Mom had a major stroke two days ago. She is unable to eat, drink, or talk. She only responds to painful stimulus."

"My wife, Iris, and I decided to bring her home and let her pass peacefully with us. The whole family is flying here today to say their goodbyes. It will be a family reunion. She would want it that way, with lots of conversation and food. No tears."

"Sara has lived independently in her home since dad died ten years ago," Dr. John continued. "We called her every morning to check on her. When she didn't answer her phone, Iris rushed to her house. She found her unconscious on the floor. Mother was cold, but alive.

The paramedics came and took her to the hospital where an MRI showed a massive CVA (cerebral vascular accident). Since that moment she has not regained consciousness. Long ago she had made me promise to let her go naturally if she had a major stroke. She did not want a feeding tube to lengthen her life or any other life saving measures."

"I have the durable power of health care (DPAHC) and will sign the consents to start hospice today."

Time was of essence for Dr. John. "Come sit down with me at the table. I have a fresh pot of coffee. Would you like a cup?

"Yes, I like it black."

Dr. John poured a cup of steaming hot coffee. We sat down at the kitchen table where about twenty sheets of paper flew under his silver pen. "Keep the back copies. I'll read them later. Thanks." He left immediately, leaving me alone with my coffee. I began to tear the patient copies from the forms and stack them neatly on the table.

After a few minutes, Iris entered the kitchen in designer jeans and a black sweatshirt. She smiled. "I'm Iris, like the flower. You must have had to get up very early this morning. Do you need to eat something? You can have a toasted bagel and cream cheese with me. Have you ever tried lox?"

I have no idea what lox is, except I know it is not for my bike or part of my hairdo.

"I'm not sure what lox is."

"Lox is raw smoked salmon. Do you like salmon?"

"I love salmon but I've never eaten it raw."

"Oh, be brave."

"Okay. I'll try it."

"We usually eat the raw salmon with cream cheese on warm toasted bagel with capers. Would you like to try capers too?"

"Why not, I'll try anything once!"

Iris smothered the fresh toasted onion bagel with cream cheese. She sprinkled capers, then pressed the lox into the cream cheese" "You can also have onions and tomatoes with it. Maybe we can add onions and tomatoes at another time."

She handed me the bagel and lox, reached for the coffee pot, and offered me another cup. Iris sat down as I tasted the delicacy.

Mm, this is good. Tastes like a breakfast fit for a Queen . . . Did Queen Esther eat like this in Babylon?

"Your husband has signed all the consent forms. He must be familiar with hospice. Let me go over some basics."

Iris set her coffee on the table. "John has shared with me what he knows about hospice. He arranged it with Sara's primary physician. I would appreciate hearing what hospice can do for Sara and the family."

Over my unusual breakfast, I started my presentation. "Hospice is a free benefit to your family because Sara is on

Medicare." Iris listened as I explained the team concept, the services hospice would provide, and the responsibilities of the caregiver.

"Sara has been admitted onto hospice. Your husband has signed all the consents, but I still need to see her social security card. Here are the back copies to read. I'll put everything in your hospice folder."

"Please call our hospice number for any questions. Your husband believes Sara's condition is life-threatening and he specified he does not want any interventions or life support. All he wants is to keep her comfortable."

"I'll make a visit every morning to make sure Sara is comfortable and see how you're doing. Is seven a.m. too early?"

"I'm up at that time. That's also good for John. He usually leaves soon after seven."

"I'll arrange for a home health aide to give Sara a bath and take care of her hygiene needs. I'll have her call you to schedule a visit. Would that be okay with you?"

"Yes, I'd be happy to have a health aide bathe Sara. I didn't think hospice would help us so much."

"Please expect a phone call from our social worker. She'll schedule a visit. I think you'll find her to be an emotional support."

"That's very important for my three teenagers. They'll need help getting through their grandmother dying in our home. They're very close to her and love her deeply. How soon can she come?"

"She'll be here later today or tomorrow. I'll have her call you. If there's any change in Sara's condition, call me. Here's a magnet with hospice's number to place on your refrigerator, stickers for your phones, and my business card."

"Would you like a hospice chaplain or do you have a rabbi?"

"We have Rabbi Joe who's already been here. Thanks for the offer."

"May I see Sara now?"

"Sure. Go ahead."

"Would you like to join me?"

"No. I need to find her social security card."

Sara is 96 years old with a long history of multiple TIA's (transit ischemic attacks), history of high blood pressure and atrial fib (irregular heart rhythm). Hmmm ... Did she throw a blood clot with her uncontrolled atrial fib?

She was unaware as I took her vital signs. I checked her skin for pressure sores and reddened areas around bony prominences. I saw numbers tattooed on her right arm.

Is Sara a Holocaust survivor?

Her mouth was dry, lips were cracked, tongue was parched, and breath smelled abnormal. Sara was dehydrated.

With my flashlight I observed fixed and dilated pupils. There was no response to light.

She's not responding because there is minimal brain activity.

While I was completing the assessment, Sara's grandchildren entered. "Who are you?"

"I'm Karen, Sara's nurse. I will be caring for your grandmother?"

"Is she going to get better?"

"Your dad told me she had a big stroke. We both agree she will not get better."

"You mean she's going to die?"

"Unless a miracle happens and she comes out of her coma, she'll leave us. She's not responding to me. She'll probably not respond to you."

"You can still talk and sing to her. I think she can still hear you. Hearing is the last sense to leave. As you lightly massage lotion on her arms and legs or comb her hair, you can tell her how much you love her."

45

"How long will you be staying with your grandmother?"

"We're not staying here. We live here! We're in and out, depending on our college class schedules."

"When you have time, keep her lips moist with Chap Stick and her tongue wet with a wet cool washrag. I have some green sponge mint toothettes to keep her mouth and teeth clean. Let me show you how." The girls watched as I got a glass of water, dipped the toothettes, and carefully wiped around her teeth and tongue. "Throw the toothettes away after each use. I will leave you a few packages."

"You can help your parents by taking shifts to turn her. You'll need to turn her every two hours. Our hospice health aide will come today and teach you how to keep her comfortable."

"Oh, it won't be necessary!" Iris had entered the living room. "John and I have hired a twenty-four hour CNA (Certified Nursing Assistant). Will you be able instruct her? She's expected to be here within the hour."

"If she arrives before I finish my visit, I will be happy to talk with her. A licensed caregiver should know how to care for her."

"Here's Sara's social security card. I found it in her jewelry box!"

Iris and I went back into the kitchen where I finished my assessment paper work and carefully copied her social security number and letters onto the consent.

When the family's paid caregiver arrived, we had a short conversation. I knew she would be able to care for Sara. She had years of hospice experience.

At the office, I penned into my schedule a daily nursing visit knowing Sara would not be with us more than a few days. She would soon be in renal failure from dehydration.

Each day I checked on Sara's condition, made sure she was comfortable, clean, and safe. I recited the Twenty-Third Psalm and quietly whispered a prayer. Then I had bagels and lox with the family. It was a special time to listen and learn about Sara, the matriarch of their family. Her three granddaughters loved their precious grandmother. They did not want her to die.

On the fourth morning I found Sara lying on her side with shallow rapid respirations. She had changed from nasal to mouth breathing. I changed the nasal cannula (plastic tubing for the nose) to an oxygen mask and increased the oxygen level to five liters per minute.

The blood pressure was impalpable. Heart rate was thready (faint), around 160. She seemed agitated. Legs were mottled (a bluish/maroon marbling skin tone) from her toes to her knees. Skin was wet with perspiration. Feet were cold. Face was pale white and lips were blue. Her diaper was dry. She was actively dying.

After reaching for the lotion at the bed side, I began to massage her back before I turned her to lie facing me. Her eyes were half open with a blank stare.

She still is not following me with her eyes. I think she's seeing someone bidding her to come. Maybe it's her mom or dad. I wish I could see what she sees.

Sara's paid caregiver helped as I laid her on her back and used the bed controls to change her position to sitting. I supported her tiny frame with pillows. Placing a pillow under her knees, I pushed the button on the remote to raise her knees to keep her in an upright position.

This will slow her respiration rate and make her comfortable. I don't think she will last another twelve hours. She needs a little more medication to help her relax.

Sara's caregiver touched me on my shoulder. "Is there anything else I need to do?"

"Continue with her medications every two hours. I'll call her doctor with an update. If the orders change, I'll call you. You don't have to turn her now. She will be less agitated if you don't. If she doesn't appear comfortable, please have Iris call me. You are doing a wonderful job and I appreciate all your help."

Before leaving I met with the family. "Sara's passing will be soon. I'll be available all day for you and 'on call' tonight. In these last hours you can talk with her. Patients often hold on to life until they know they have permission to leave. Tell her it's okay. She needs your permission to let go. It will be easier for her."

A tear started down Iris' cheek. I reached my arms out to embrace her. "I am so sorry, Iris."

"It's been very hard. Mom's my best friend and I am having a very difficult time saying good-bye. The embrace lasted until she loosed her hug.

"I hope at the end of my life I'll have someone to care for me like we have done for Sara."

"Will Dr. John be coming home early today?"

"Yes, he told me he was leaving the office at noon. He knows mom probably will not last through the day. We'll call if we need you."

"I'll keep in touch with you."

Around ten-thirty I called Iris. "Mom looks comfortable. John's coming home in an hour. I'll have him call you when he gets here."

"I spoke with Sara's doctor. You can double the dose of Roxanol so she can breathe easier. Give her one milliliter of Roxanol every two hours under her tongue."

During my lunch break the office connected me with Dr. John. "Mother's heart rate is one hundred seventy-eight. She's clammy and in Cheyne Stokes (shallow irregular breathing)."

"Is she comfortable?"

"I hope so. Maybe I should give her another dose of Ativan."

"When was the last time it was given?"

"Hold on. Let me check." The phone went silent for a moment. "About two hours ago."

"Go ahead and give her another dose of two milligrams under her tongue. Remember to crush it in a teaspoon and add a few drops of warm water to dissolve it. Follow it with one milliliter of Roxanol with the eye dropper. Would you like me to come and be with you?"

"No, it's not necessary. I wanted you to be aware of her condition. I don't think it will be much longer. The family's here. We're doing alright. Thanks for preparing the girls."

"I think she's ending her life's marathon. Call me back in forty minutes if the medication hasn't helped."

It was less than an hour when the office again connected us. Iris calmly said, "She's finally at peace. She stopped breathing."

"I'll be there in twenty minutes."

"Take your time. Be safe. I know God's malakh is with you. There is no hurry now. Come when your can."

"Is malakh an angel in Hebrew?"

"Yes, it's an angel, God's messenger."

"Is there anything I can do?"

"No. The waiting is over. Her battle for life is finished."

"By the way, we're happy you were Sara's nurse. There's no way we can repay you for your kindness. Thank you."

When I reached their home I found the family around her bedside listening to Jewish music. The CNA was washing Sara's face. I walked to Sara's bedside and confirmed she was no longer breathing. I looked at Iris standing by my side. "I'm glad she's in a better place. Maybe she flew on the wings of her malakh."

"I hope you're right, Karen."

Dr. John stood up and came to my side. "I was with mom when she died. Holding her hand, I told her it was okay to leave. She seemed to understand, took a deep sigh, and she was gone. I've already called the mortuary and they'll be here soon."

The family was quietly sitting around the living room eating fresh salad, fruit, bagels, and lox. I looked at Dr. John. "We're planning mom's funeral and reminiscing the good times we had together.'

How blessed to be able to enjoy the good times spent with Sara.

One of the granddaughters stood up and took me by my hand into the family room. "Let me show you a picture of Grandmother Sara when she was young." She pointed to a black and white photo of her as a child in Lithuania before the Holocaust and one on the day she was married. On the other wall was a gallery of Sara's ten grandchildren and nineteen great grandchildren. In the center of the gallery was a 16 x 20 inch gold framed picture with Sara proudly sitting on a tall chair in the middle.

She's beautiful.

Before I left, I discarded the narcotics and asked Dr. John if he wanted to keep the remaining medications.

"What good would they be to me? You can get rid of them."

The family invited me to the funeral the following afternoon.

I've never been to a Jewish funeral.

The funeral service was at the local synagogue where Sara worshiped. I attended the service and took a single red rose to give to the family. It was a symbol of my love for them.

As I walked across the parking lot, I was surprised, when a friend of the family approached me. "We never have flowers at our funerals. Please, keep it for yourself."

"Thank you for telling me. I'll put it back in my car." Embarrassed I hurried to my car and laid the rose on the seat. A tear came to my eye and trickled down my cheek.

I should have given it to Sara when she was still alive. Could she have smelled it?

I exchanged the rose for a sympathy card from my collection in the glove compartment. I wrote the words of the twenty-third Psalm from the Holy Scriptures:

"The Lord is my shepherd; I shall not want. He makes me lie down in green pastures; He leads me beside the still waters. He restores my soul; He leads me in the paths of righteousness for His name sake.

Even though I walk through the valley of the shadow of death, I will fear no evil; for you are with me; your rod and your staff, they comfort me.

You prepare a table for me in the presence of my enemies; you anoint my head with oil; my cup runs over.

Surely goodness and mercy shall follow me all the days of my life and I will dwell in the house of the Lord forever."

With the addition of "I'll be praying for you," I signed the card, "Love, your nurse Karen, who really loves bagels and lox. Shalom."

Sara had lived a long life full of faith. Those who knew her respected and adored her.

Following the service I told the family, "I'm going to miss those delicious bagels. Thank for introducing me to lox and cream cheese. I might make it a habit to eat bagels and lox to remember Sara and you."

A week after the funeral I called Iris and reminded her our grief counselor was available.

"That would be wonderful. Death was traumatic for all of us, especially for our girls. I'm not sure how to help them. I don't know what to say. When can she come?"

"I'll have our grief counselor call and schedule a time to start."

Grieving will be hard work. It will not get better with time. They will grieve as deeply as they loved.

When they grieve, it will be because part of their heart went with their grandmother. Their wound will take time to heal. The scar that forms will last their whole life. When music or a smell reminds them of her, it will bring an emotional heart felt response, usually followed by a tear or a lump in their throat.

When the grief counselor met with the granddaughters, she provided time to listen and share their feelings. During the next year she took the girls through the stages of grieving: denial, anger, bargaining, depression, and acceptance. She provided them with materials to read, and encouraged them to write a letter to their grandmother.

Elisabeth Kubler Ross is the pioneer for grieving. Thank you, Elizabeth.

Four months after Sara's passing, Dr. John called. He thanked me for the hospice team's support. He asked how he could make a donation. I told him he could send it to our hospice address.

"Dr. John, thank you for your kindness. You introduced me to fresh bagels, soft cream cheese and lox, a new tradition."

This time the early bird didn't get a worm. She got bagels and lox, plus capers! What an experience!

SHALOM
Peace with God
Marge Anselma

How good to know that God above,
Fills us daily with His love.
So great that it will never cease,
To fill our hearts with perfect peace.

When trying circumstances prevail,
And all our efforts are to no avail,
We struggle and cry, then we finally pray;
And experience God's peace, which is there to stay.

The world wants peace instead of war.
But they don't understand what they're fighting for.
Before peace can reign in the outermost parts,
God's 'Shalom' must fill our hearts.

(Used with permission of the author)

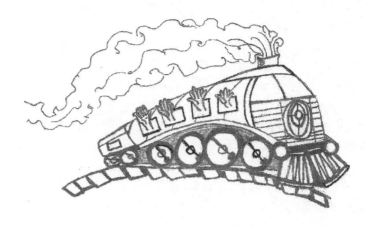

GET ON BOARD

It was pouring rain as I put the address of my newest hospice patient into my GPS. It said eight point two miles to the destination in the middle of the city where the poorest of the poor lived out their existence. It was a gang ghetto area where houses looked like run down shacks.

Guess I should have joined a martial arts class years ago

My nursing supervisor told me to watch my back and be alert.

I'll take a minute to look carefully at my surroundings and pray before I unlock my door.

I drove a red Mustang convertible with RNKAREN for a license plate.

I believe I have angels guarding me. I remember seeing two of them at different times. I hope they're on duty today.

My patient was living in his meager small, one bedroom apartment filled with old magazines, lots of books, and dirty dishes piled high on the kitchen counter.

His legal name was Anthony, but his doctor told me to call him Tony. He lived alone, a real bachelor, since his wife died years before.

He had only one mission in life. It was to live long enough to make sure all his grandchildren were 'living right.'

His face changed as he shook his head. "I've given up on some of my own kids, they have made poor choices; but all my grandchildren need to 'get on board.'"

On board, hmm ... what does that mean?

He was tall and thin in stature. I could see every bone in his body.

There are usually two hundred six bones in the human body! He's a good specimen for an anatomy class.

"Nothing I eat tastes good any more. I need a new tongue! I miss those old days when I was a child in Alabama. I would come into the house and smell my mom's black eyed peas cooking on the stove and the cornbread baking in her old brick oven. Those were the days when I could eat lots of food and never gain a pound!"

"I guess remembering them is better than doing them. Picking cotton from dawn till dusk wasn't fun, but it sure gives you an appetite," he told me, laughingly. "You should have seen me when I was working in those fields. I weighed one hundred seventy-eight pounds of pure muscle."

Tony's primary care doctor was also our hospice director. At one of our hospice team meetings, he told us about Tony's declining condition. "He has end stage esophageal cancer, metastasized to both lungs. He's an insulin dependent diabetic with a weak heart. He has refused a feeding tube for nourishment and said he wanted to die at home. He's really tired of frequent ER visits and hospitalizations."

After explaining what hospice meant, Tony thought hospice care might help him. He stared at me and said, "I'll sign the papers if you'll always be my nurse."

"I can be your case manager, but there is no guarantee someone else from my office might make a visit. That would only happen if I were sleeping or sick. Remember, when I am not working there is always a nurse on call. We take turns being on duty during the weekends and nights."

After answering all his questions, I explained the rules of hospice. "You always call our hospice number first. You never call nine-one-one. You must be home when a member of the hospice team schedules a visit. You must keep your house safe for yourself and us."

"Suits me fine!"

"We also have a chaplain. Are you interested?"

"Not really. My pastor is a close friend. He'll be happy to visit me anytime I call. My church is around the corner. Here, look out my window. Can you see the cross?"

"Yes, it's beautiful. Does it light up at night?"

"Yes it does. I see it every evening and morning. I gain strength for the day knowing the cross is there."

Tony signed on the bottom line. He understood he could request to stop hospice at any time. If his condition improved, hospice would discharge him.

Tony got 'on board,' but, in my heart, I knew it would not be very long before he would leave this world for a place without cancer, pain, or tears. I hoped he had time to get his grandchildren 'on board,' as he put it.

Tony was seventy-five years old. He had been a professional baseball player in his younger days, still loved baseball, and was an avid Dodger fan. He watched every game the Dodgers played and knew every player's name, position, averages, and salaries.

He always wore his tattered royal blue Dodger cap with the logo 'LA Dodgers' in dingy white.

I need to wash that cap or exchanged it for a new one. Maybe I can get him one for Christmas and fill it with Skittles and M&M's. He would love sharing them with his grandkids.

His ten grandsons and six granddaughters had nick-named him 'Pops.' Pops was a great nickname because he loved his nightly popcorn when he could swallow without pain. They all enjoyed watching baseball games together, but their best memories were learning to play baseball in the sandlot with Pops as their coach.

Tony also loved to read books. He told me the Bible was his favorite. "I wish I understood more about how the Bible predicts the world will end. I read the Bible every morning. It's my daily bread."

"When I'm alone, I like to read the Bible out loud. I'm getting to the place where I run out of breath when I do that."

He always left his Bible open on his king sized bed along with three old soft blue pillows and his cat.

"Midnight is black and I'm black. The big difference is Midnight can purr, I can only pant!" I laughed. He had a great sense of humor.

"Tony, what's going to happen to Midnight when you die?"

"Oh, one of the kids will take him. If not, they'll let him go and he'll find his own home. That's what he did to find me. He meowed so loud I had to feed him!"

Tony asked me a burning question. "What happens when we die? I'm ready whenever my Maker calls me, but I'm not sure how it works, since I haven't done it before!"

Sitting down on the end of his double bed I asked him, "Have you taken the time to read the blue booklet in your hospice folder called *Gone from My Sight*?"

He was proud to tell me, "I have read all the materials in my folder, but reading something in a book isn't like doing it." I smiled.

He's got a good point, he's right!

For Tony, I explained the dying process in baseball terms.

"Tony, dying is like playing a game of baseball. When you round all the bases and touch home plate, you're finished, right?"

He nodded his head and replied, "Especially if it's the bottom of the ninth, and you're tied!"

Then I held his hand. "When you were diagnosed with cancer and completed all your treatments, your life expectancy was six months. That gave you a walk to first base." I touched his index finger.

"When your body can no longer walk without the help of a walker or cane, you steal second base." I touched his second finger.

Tony piped up, "Well, I guess I'm on second base, right?"

"Yep, you're on second base. When you are bed bound, you have advanced to third base."

I gently placed three of his fingers in my hand and held them. "Waiting on third base before heading to home plate might seem like forever, lying in bed.

The time will come when you can no longer swallow food or fluids. This usually lasts only three to four days. The kidneys stop working and you begin the long walk to home plate."

I slowly closed all his fingers in my hand. "Because of dehydration, your heart will start beating hard and very fast, and it will stop when the kidneys can't get rid of the waste products from your body. During this time you will be sleeping and someone will keep you comfortable with the medications the doctor will order."

Smiling at him I said, "When you start to leave third base you will need someone to stay with you twenty four hours a day. This is your slow walk home."

Tony opened his hand and took mine with both of his. He said with tears mounting in his big brown eyes, "I have no one except my homeless friend, who cares enough to check on me every day. He may be able to help me."

"Your friend would be a great baseline coach to help you reach home plate."

Tony smiled. "I'll have him here to meet you next Thursday, when you come. Could you tell Frank what you told me? I've known him for a couple of years."

"Yes, I'll be happy to explain everything to him."

On the next visit I met Frank. The discussion of hospice went far better than I expected. Frank was happy to have a place to stay out of the rain and chilly foggy weather. Even though he had no nursing experience, Frank was willing to care for him when the time came for Tony to walk to home plate.

Tony was a good sport as I taught Frank how to turn and diaper him. I explained how important it was to keep Tony dry and clean. Both Tony and I were surprised how quickly Frank learned these skills.

Half of my job is teaching.

Some of his sixteen grandchildren dropped in to visit Pops every week. Tony made sure they all knew the way to heaven on each visit. This was his way of 'getting them on board.'

He decided to write his own eulogy when he was still on second base, and still had the energy. He picked out the Bible passages he wanted read, the songs he wanted sung, and even asked me to record him singing his favorite song, the old spiritual *Get on Board Little Chillun*.

"Karen, do you ever have any special dreams?"

"I dream, but usually can't remember all the details unless it's a special dream."

"Last night, I saw a train with all my grandkids hanging out of the windows singing. I tried counting noses, but I couldn't see their faces, just their hands. I think they all have made the train bound for glory. I've talked to every one of them. I want to be there at heaven's gate to welcome them home. I know this, my wife is there wondering what's taking me so long!"

Tony is dreaming, like many of my patients. They often dream of their parents, children, or friends who have already died. Tony's dream is an exception. He's dreaming of his living grandchildren. He must love them dearly.

The time came when Tony moved to third base. He was too weak to walk. I ordered a hospital bed with an alternating air pressure mattress.

He was unable to get out of the bed. He refused all soft food. Water became too difficult to swallow. He could only suck on crushed ice chips for fluids.

It was time for Frank to put his training into practice. He slept on his army cot next to Tony, who had been his chess partner for years. They both knew what it was like to lose their queen in a match, or call out, 'check mate' on the king. But neither one knew had how hard it would be to say, 'check-mate,' in real life. Tony was losing his game of life. Tony's check-mate would leave Frank behind.

No one should expect one person to be a twenty-four hour caregiver while a patient walks to home plate. The caregiver needs to turn and medicate the patient every two hours. Frank was fifty years old. He apparently thought he could take care of Tony twenty-four/seven. He soon realized he could not get enough sleep, and became exhausted

He's fried. He needs more sleep. SOS social worker!

The social worker visited Tony, and offered a hospice respite. Hospice could place Pops in a facility for one week, all expenses paid. After his week of respite, he would return home or be admitted into a facility. Tony could not afford a facility unless it would settle for his monthly social security check.

One of Tony's granddaughters overheard the conversation. She made another suggestion. "We can be with Pops during the day and Frank can be with him during the night. We can work it out, no problem."

Three granddaughters were free to care for Pops in the day hours. They seemed happy to help.

They quickly learned how to turn and diaper him. I also taught them how to give his pain medications, reposition him, and give oral care.

They were able to reposition Pops and keep him dry and clean every two or three hours. This prevented bed sores.

They told me they pretended they were blind and always put a hand towel over his private areas.

Modesty at its greatest!

Two of the girls told me they were going to study nursing to become RN's.

I hope I am an inspiration.

A hospice home health aide gave Tony a bath every other day, changed the linens, and was an emotional support to the granddaughters.

With six to seven hours of sleep during the day, Frank was able to stay awake through the night, the toughest shift. He was truly a 'homeless earth angel' who loved strong black coffee!

Frank is earning his pair of angel wings with honor! He is a remarkable man, a faithful friend.

The grandchildren dropped in on Pops often and sang his favorite spirituals. Even his own children came to visit and love him.

Bright and early Friday morning, I stood at the old unpainted front door. I could hear the sound of a grandchildren's gospel choir. I waited for a few minutes, lost in the melody, with tears rolling down my cheeks.

How I love Tony and his family. They make being a nurse worthwhile and make me thankful for this opportunity to help Tony arrive at home plate. I'm sure Tony can hear their praises.

The singing stopped. I knocked loudly on the door, no one heard me. I rang the doorbell, no one came. I slowly opened the door and found everyone laughing and talking loudly around the kitchen table. They were eating a southern breakfast of grits, bacon, and coffee.

"Want some breakfast Karen?"

"No thanks. How's Pops?"

"He's doing the same. Sleeps most of the time."

After talking with the grandchildren, I walked over to Tony's bed. He looked like he had run a hundred miles. I could hear his labored breathing. He was wet with sweat, non-responsive to touch, was wearing his oxygen mask, and had bluish hands, legs, and feet.

His grandchildren had positioned him on his left side with pillows sticking out from his body in every direction. I smiled knowing they were loving him in the best way they knew.

Sitting beside Tony, I held his hand and whispered a prayer in his ear.

I hollered loudly, "Can someone come and help me turn Tony onto his back?"

"Sure, we'll be right there."

With the bed's remote, I lowered the head of the bed to the lowest position and raised his bed to the level of my waist. When help arrived, we turned him on his back and with the draw sheet gently lifted him to the top of the bed.

He will be touching home plate soon.

He was breathing in short shallow irregular breaths.

He looks like a fish out of water trying to suck in water so he could get enough oxygen to live.

Taking the bottle of Roxanol, I gave Tony a dose under his tongue.

His mouth is dry and parched.

Raising my hand, I tried to get the attention of the rest of Tony's grandchildren. "Tony's about ready to take his high

63

speed train to glory." I motioned for them. "Come over here so we can be together as he leaves for heaven."

"Go wake Frank up," someone yelled.

The room became quiet and the grandchildren came over to his bedside. Each one laid a hand on his cold body, bowed their heads, and I heard them begin to pray. Frank squeezed in and leaned over my shoulder.

We are family now.

Frank and I were holding Tony's cold hands. With the prayers in the background, I put my lips to his ear. "Tony, it's time to let go and slide into home plate. You know all your grandchildren are 'on board.' They're on the train now. It's time to let go."

The grandchildren stopped praying and started telling Pops good-bye.

"Good-bye Pops. It's okay to go."

"I will always feel your presence with me. I love you."

"Go find Nana, tell her hi for us. I will always love you, Pops."

"Tell Jesus, 'hi' for me."

As his family continued to say good-bye, he took his last gasp of air. He was gone from his body. His spirit and soul left to a new world. He was free from cancer. No more suffering. He went peacefully to his God.

I feel those wings again dancing around me at this sacred moment of exchanging places from earth to heaven. It must be exhilarating to fly so high so fast!

The family joined hands, stood around Tony, and asked me to lead in prayer. I tried, but my tears got in the way of my words. I heard the family lifting their voices to their heavenly Father, praying their Pops would enjoy his ride into heaven and find Nana, their grandmother.

There were several 'Amens.'

A granddaughter began to sing a beautiful song, one I had not heard before. Soon all the grandchildren were singing.

Over the sunset ocean,
Someday I'll quickly go,
Into the arms of my Savior,
The one who has loved me so.

Over the sunset ocean,
Our Savior waits for me.
Over the sunset ocean,
With Him forever I'll be.

"Ms. Karen, don't you know a heaven song we can sing?"
"How about singing Amazing Grace?"
They all joined in:

Amazing Grace how sweet the sound
That saved a wretch like me.
I once was lost, but now am found,
Was blind, but now I see.

"Let me teach you a new way to sing the last verse. Instead of ten thousand years, we'll sing ten million years." I started to sing. All of the grandchildren joined me in beautiful harmony.

When we've been there ten million years,
Bright shining as the sun.
There's no less days to sing God' praise,
Than when we've first begun.

Angels are singing and dancing all around us. I can feel their presence!
"Would you like me to give Pops his last bath?"
"No way! He wouldn't want you to work another minute. He isn't here anymore, he's with Jesus."

When the family was ready, I called the necessary numbers to take Tony's body to the mortuary. When the white van arrived everyone wanted to kiss him goodbye, one last time, and tell him how much they loved him. They all told him they would miss eating popcorn, watching baseball, and even going to church with him.

When the doorbell rang, the two grandsons looked at me and asked, "Can we carry Pops to the van?" These two grandsons could have been NFL linemen. I knew they could lift Pops, He only weighed ninety-five pounds.

I don't think they'll drop him, but if they're not careful, they could hurt themselves. If they drop him, it wouldn't be very dignified. It would be a very bad memory!

Smiling at them, "Go ahead, be careful."

The oldest grandson bent over and wrapped an old tattered red blanket tightly around Pops. He lifted him into his arms, held him close to his heart, and carried him to the van.

One of the other grandsons whispered to me, "Remember he's not heavy, he's our Pops! I wish I had been the oldest so I could have carried him. That would have been a special honor."

After they placed Tony's body on a gurney and slid him into the van, we held hands and sang Pop's favorite song. *Get on board Little Chilluns.* We changed the words to say,

We're on board little chilluns,
We're on board little chilluns,
We're on board little chilluns,
There's room for many a more!"

Missing Tony's memorial service was not an option. I rearranged my schedule so I could attend.

Tony's pastor officiated. He had made several visits to see Tony during the three months he was on hospice. In his message he said Tony had told him all of his grandchildren

66

were 'on the train bound for glory.' Now they were brothers and sisters in God's big family.

The service was not sad, but rather a celebration of his life and homecoming to heaven's open gate. I cried when I heard my recording of his voice singing his song:

Get on Board little Chillun,
Get on Board little Chillun,
Get on Board little Chillun,
There's room for many a more."

All of his eight children attended his memorial service. They took turns telling their hilarious stories of Pops. When the service was almost over, they asked me to speak. I felt honored.

My knees are shaking and I can't think of what to say. I should have written something down on a three by five card!

"Thank you for the honor of being Tony's hospice nurse." I started to cry and all I could say was, "I loved him."

Six of his oldest grandsons were pallbearers, and I knew they were singing in their hearts as they walked the long church aisle, "He ain't heavy, he's our Pops." They carried the simple pine box with pride and dignity wearing their best suits and colorful ties. As they passed me, they smiled and gave me a wink.

I understood their wink.

I gave them my biggest smile and winked back.

Today, Tony's up in heaven waiting for his grandchildren. He'll get to see them 'on board,' each time the train to glory stops for one of them. As for his children, I think they'll make it too.

As I left the church parking lot, I started singing Tony's song.

'Get on board little chillun will always be a part of my heart and remind me of Tony. ... Oh no, I didn't get to buy him a new Dodger ball cap! Is there baseball in heaven?

Tony's grandchildren were there to say good-bye when he died. The dying need their family and friends in those last days to say farewell.

Along with good-bye, the simple words, 'I love you,' work every time.

But as many as received Him to them gave He power to become the sons of God, even to them that believe on His name.   John 1:12 (KJV)

SOMETIMES
Karen Farr
2015

Sometimes we wonder why
Life seems but a vapor,
Or a tiny flower fading
In the heat of the sun.

A miracle to start life
At a baby's first cry,
But too quickly gone,
And then wonder why.

Live life as a fragile gift
From the good Lord above,
Knowing you can never open it
Without faith in our Father's love.

Sometimes we can share the gift
Of life eternal to those lost along the way,
Hold their hand and say a prayer
For God to show them His perfect way.

RICHES
Howard Ellowis
2015

How do we define them?
When do they take place?

They begin with the day.
We transfer from sleep to wakefulness
The first thing we see,
The first thought we have,
The first movement we make,
We explode into being,
We rocket into life.

Life itself is the greatest riches of all!

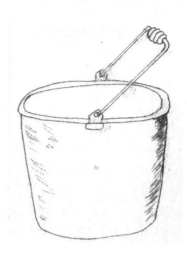

THE ORANGE BUCKET

A hospice phone never stops ringing! I intercepted a front office call and spoke to a frantic daughter asking to talk to someone about getting help for her dad. "I live in the city, and my dad's living alone in the desert. He has terminal lung cancer. He smoked a pack a day of Marlboros, most of his life. He has tried all the chemo and radiation treatments available, but nothing has helped. His oncologist gave me your number."

Terminal is not in my vocabulary, unless I'm talking about an airport. Life threatening sounds a lot better to me.

After a few words of emotional support, I transferred her call to our admitting nurse. She spoke with her to verify the patient's address, phone number, and doctor's name. The admitting nurse would call his oncologist and ask if he would fax an admit order.

The referral landed on my desk by the end of the day.

This is the daughter I spoke with this morning.

Since the community where her dad lived was in my area, my nursing supervisor assigned Gary to me. After reading his medical chart, I decided to phone Gary's daughter to arrange a convenient time to join her dad for a possible admission.

"Hello, Betty?"

"Yes. Who's calling?"

"This is Karen, from the hospice office you called this morning."

"I remember your voice. I'm glad you called me back."

"You're the daughter I spoke with this morning. How are you?"

"Not so good. Dad is really sick. I hope you can help him."

"Will you be caring for him?"

"Not really. I'm his Durable Power of Health Care, but I'm only responsible if there is an emergency. I'd like to hear about hospice, but it's really his decision."

"His oncologist faxed a referral order to start his care. I would like you to join me at your father's home."

"Yes, I can make arrangements to be there."

"I see you live an hour or more from him. Is he aware of your call to hospice?"

"Yes, he asked me to call. It's not easy to do this for him. We don't have a good relationship. We're on speaking terms now, only because he has cancer. We have many differences. The biggest is our religion. He's New Age and I'm Mormon."

"Can we meet this Friday at one? That'll give you time to travel."

"Friday at one will be fine. I'll call dad and tell him. He lives in an unfinished house. Being a bachelor, he doesn't care!"

It was almost one when I arrived at Gary's home. His house was a work in progress. There was a silver Toyota Camry and a large camper in the driveway. Scaffolds, ladders, an old compressor, and an orange tractor littered the rocky front yard. The tall columns on the front porch were unpainted. The garage door was open and I saw an old red Honda parked inside.

Climbing up three stairs between empty five gallon paint cans, I landed safely on an unfinished plywood porch. I pressed the doorbell on the unpainted door jam. Nothing happened. I pressed it again. There was no sound. I knocked on the door several times. No response.

Betty said she'd call her dad. No one's answering the door. Strange. I'll try calling Gary on my cell phone.

As I was returning to my car to make the call, a male voice yelled from the garage, "My door bell doesn't work and the front door doesn't open. Come on in through the garage. Friends always use the garage entrance, right?"

"Okay. I'll be right there, Gary."

He must see me as a friend already. Just wait until his first enema!

The garage was a maze of ladders, motorcycles, auto parts, empty paint cans, old oil spills, and overflowing trash cans alongside a classic red nineteen seventy-six Honda in primo condition.

A bachelor's paradise! Hope I can make it without breaking my leg.

I zigged zagged through the garage and stepped into the house. Betty helped me step around a saw horse. Gary was already heading down the hallway as I stepped into the house. Betty walked behind me as I followed Gary to the kitchen between stacks of tile boxes and buckets of adhesive.

The kitchen cupboards were without doors. On the shelves were a few paper plates, Styrofoam cups and an empty paper towel role. A dripping faucet stood over a large bowl perched on a step stool.

He has running water from the faucet. Does someone have to run outside to empty the bowl of water? Wow, that is running water!

The sink was sitting on the floor.

I hope he hires someone to install the sink.

A greasy old frying pan was still on the stove half filled with thick white bacon grease. Resting on the Formica counter top, still rough around the edges, was a juicer surrounded by wilted collards, kale, celery, and spinach.

Oh my! Is this a nightmare or is this for real?

Gary was sitting at the kitchen table and pointing at two folding chairs. "There's room to sit here."

Betty and I smiled at each other and took his advice.

Betty started the conversation. "Gary, this is Karen. She's here to explain hospice."

"Nice to meet you, Karen. Don't mind this house. I've been building it for the past three years. I started before my third wife left me. It's only partially finished, as you can see, but it's good enough for an old bachelor like me!"

Gary is sixty-seven years old, appearing to be strong, but failing in his fight with cancer.

"Gary, can you share you medical history?"

"I have survived two rounds of chemotherapy over six months and I still have excruciating headaches, upper back pain, nausea, and vomiting. I don't know if it's from the cancer or from the treatment."

"What has your doctor told you?"

"He said continuing with chemo treatments wouldn't make any difference, since the cancer has spread to my brain and bones. There's no hope, no medical cure."

"I understand."

"Why is this happening to me."

"I wish I had the answer to that question. This I do know, our hospice team will support you wherever and as long as you live." I continued to present the guidelines of hospice and services our hospice could provide.

After listening to Gary's concerns and answering his questions, he decided to 'try' hospice to see if it could help him with his symptoms.

My physical assessment verified his diagnosis. His cancer diagnosis and willingness to stop all medical treatments made him eligible for hospice.

Betty witnessed him signing the hospice consent forms. Gary agreed not to call nine-one-one for any emergency. Instead he would phone the hospice number for any problems.

"Gary, a hospice nurse will be on call twenty four hours a day and seven days a week. The on-call nurse will be able to help you by phone or make a visit, if needed"

Gary agreed to having two nursing visits a week.

On the third visit, I found Gary gone. His new camper was gone. I called our social worker and reported him as missing. She advised me to wait three days until the next scheduled visit before we made a 'missing person's report.' She suggested a daily phone call to his home.

My phone calls and messages went unanswered. It became mandatory to make another visit to his home.

His camper was in the driveway.

Believe it or not, he's here!

"Where have you been, Gary?"

"I went for a little ride in the desert for some peace and quiet. I enjoy meditation and yoga, especially the Joshua trees at sunset. No one disturbs me when I listen to music or do my channeling. I'm getting enlightened."

"I didn't get a call from you telling me you wouldn't be home! If it happens again we will have to take you off hospice. Being absent on a planned visit without any notice means something is wrong and we are required to report you as missing. By the way, when you signed the 'Rights and Responsibilities' consent, you agreed to let us know when you were going to be unavailable for a visit. You violated your agreement!"

"I forgot. You know I have brain cancer!"

What a lame brain excuse, if you ask me.

"Please, don't do it again."

"I'll do better. I'll let you know when I'm going to be traveling. I didn't think I was that important!"

"Gary, I want you to have fun doing what you love most. Enjoy life in your camper as long as you can. But keep me informed of your travels so I won't waste my time driving to your house and worrying about you."

The next time he had plans, Gary remembered to call. "I'm going to take a two week vacation all by myself. Don't plan on visiting me. I'm going to do a lot of meditating and rabbit shooting."

"Remember to bring me home a rabbit's foot," I said in jest. I notified the hospice team of his plans on our daily report line.

Two weeks without a visit? I hope he knows what he's doing!

On my first visit after he returned from his 'short' vacation, he was eager to show his pictures. "These are the sunsets and sunrises I shot while I was meditating."

"I used to be able to shoot jack rabbits. I've even shot coyotes in the desert. This time I did all my shooting with my camera. I'm too weak to hold the gun steady. My right eye, which I use to focus my scope, is now blurred. I guess my shooting days are over."

Glancing around the empty living room, I fixed my eyes on a big redwood gun case. Gary saw me looking at his gun collection and pointed his index finger like a gun to his head. "I could end all this suffering in an instant. Boom! It would be all over!"

"No more pain! Who'd care? Certainly, not my daughter!"

He knew he had shocked me. He whispered, "Don't worry. I'm too chicken to blow my head off. I might miss, and what a mess that would be."

Gary's forgotten about the rabbit's foot. I don't want a dead bunny foot dangling with my keys! That would be bad luck for me!

Gary was full of piss and vinegar. He loved to hang out with his buddies next door and talk about their hunting experiences. He was an entrepreneur, talented as a contractor, and had built many beautiful homes in the community. He had done well and had no financial concerns.

He did have a concern about dying. "If I have to die, I want to die in my own house. Is that possible?"

"Yes, if you remain safe in your home and have a caregiver a few months before you die. Do you realize you will have to hire someone to stay with you when that time comes?"

"I don't think so! If I'm unable to walk, I'll still be able to take my medications? You'll 'pack' 'em, I'll take 'em. I can manage. Think about it, Karen!"

"Gary, when you are unable to walk, you're bed bound. You won't be able to prepare your food, take your medication on time, get a glass of water, or even walk to the bathroom. As your cancer progresses, you will have difficulty in swallowing, won't be able to see clearly, and will be unable to put your medications in your mouth. It is imperative you have a caregiver at that time."

'No man's an island,' especially at the time of death.

"Do you know some pretty young girl who could help me out? She can even lay in bed with me to keep me warm, like King David."

"I don't know one, off hand. But I'll keep my eyes and ears open."

"Seriously, I always thought I would overcome the cancer because I have overcome every other obstacle in my life! Before the cancer treatment, I was a strong man, a vegetarian. I only ate healthy foods: kale, Brussels sprouts, sweet potatoes, beets, and red beans."

"When I found out I had cancer, I tried other remedies. I thought they would cure my cancer. I've tried colon therapy, lymphatic massages, and ion foot cleansing, no sugar or gluten. All of it seemed to help a little, but not enough."

"I'm doing my best to stay alive. Somewhere I learned if you drink your own urine it would cure your cancer. I am even giving it a try." Gary reached for a glass of yellow water and took several swallows. "You kind of get used to the taste."

Tell me this isn't happening. He's drinking his warm urine right in front of me. Yuk, it almost makes this nurse sick.

"It's sterile, you know. I'm also trying to limit my sugar intake. I'm still a vegetarian eating ten servings of green vegetables a day. My Nutrabullet makes great greenies. I do have one vice, ice cream. I limit my vanilla ice cream to one quart a day!"

"There's a lot of sugar in ice cream."

"I know. But you have to have at least one other vice besides smoking. I'm also taking shark cartilage in capsule form. I order it on the web. I take it every day. Anything's worth a try!"

He looked at me over his sunglasses. "Do you juice?"

"I've juiced carrots. I drank so much carrot juice my skin was turning orange."

"You have to juice other vegetables with the carrots. You should juice fruits and vegetables together. They are alkaline. Lemons, asparagus, green beans, beets, anything green is best. You need to keep your body alkaline."

Gary was trying to stay alive at all costs. His multiplying cancer cells were slowing him down in spite of his heroic attempts. He was losing two pounds a week.

In two months, Gary remembered we had a hospice chaplain and requested a visit.

"That chaplain you sent was very narrow minded. He wasn't familiar with any of my books, especially those by Helen Schucman and Deepak Chopra. He probably would never read them. He only reads the Good Book."

"He certainly has a different concept of the afterlife. He was unfamiliar with my belief about reaching a higher consciousness after death. He said he would do some research. Do you think he will?

"Yes, I think he will. I hope he's able to help you."

"He quoted several interesting things from the Bible. Maybe I should read it. It would be too hard for me to read now. I don't even own a Bible. Could you find me one?"

Our chaplain helped me find a Bible which had large print. Gary said he was able to read it with a magnifying glass.

Does he really read it? I'll ask the chaplain to read it to him.

One day Gary stopped at an auto repair shop, off the main highway, where he found someone who had survived lung cancer through three rounds of chemo. Gary had only completed two. He was convinced another round would cure him.

With this new information he made an appointment with his oncologist. After discussing his options, he decided to try a third round. He hoped 'the third time would be a charm.'

Gary contacted me and asked hospice to discharge him. He was willing to sign a planned hospice discharge consent to stop his care. This meant he would start driving forty minutes into town, three times a week, for another series of chemo-therapy treatments. For Gary it was his 'last-ditch effort.'

It was only three weeks into his chemotherapy, when he decided the side effects of nausea and vomiting, increased dizziness, and unbearable pain were worse than dying. He called our hospice office and asked if he could talk to me.

"Karen, it's not working. I feel worse than ever. Please, can you get me back on hospice?"

This time he was finished with chemotherapy!

Hospice required him to resign all of the consents as if he was starting new.

Symptom management started all over again! I called for orders to relieve the vomiting related to his recent chemotherapy, the intense head pain from his brain cancer, and his unbearable back pain. He rated his symptoms as a nine on a scale of one to ten.

One sick discouraged guy!

Now he was willing to follow my directions to stop his pain and vomiting. The doctor ordered a new prescription of decadron to decrease the swelling around his brain. His head pain went from a nine to a four.

Still need to lessen his pain. I'll call the doctor.

We had to double his regular pain medication and double his laxatives. He took the medication around the clock and it seemed he was feeling a little better every day.

We resumed our twice a week visits until he complained of not being able to catch his breath. I increased the visits to three times a week.

"Gary, you need to start using oxygen. In order to do this you must stop your habit of smoking."

"I'm not giving up one of my only vises. "I'd rather die than quit smoking!"

The three weekly visits were working out well until once again I found him missing from his home.

Oh no, he forgot to call me. I think he needs a GPS monitor on his boot! Has he wandered off into the desert with one of his guns for instant relief of pain or is he out traveling again?

His camper was in the driveway. The garage door was down. I checked the side door to the garage and it was locked.

Does his neighbor know where he may have gone?

I walked next door to check with his neighbor, who watered his trees and plants. He was clueless about Gary's whereabouts, but he had a key to the side door.

When we opened the door, his classic red Honda was missing. Gary had left in his car. He had vanished again and there was no way to contact him. He did not have a cell phone.

His daughter! Maybe she knows where he is.

I called her immediately on my cell phone.

My lucky day! Betty's number's in my Black-berry.

She answered my call. "Dad's with me and the kids. Sorry, I forgot to ask him if he had called you."

What a relief to find my lost patient.

"Dad drove here in his Honda. He gave it to Mike who turned sixteen last week. Mike is in seventh heaven with his grandfather's old car. He told me it was a classic, too good to be true!"

Later that day Betty called me back. She sounded excited. "Dad's willing to stay with us. We haven't lived together for over twenty-five years."

I notified the team of his changed address and our social worker made the appropriate arrangements for hospice care to continue with his daughter.

This was the second time he had left our hospice. The next week I made a follow-up phone call to check on my former runaway patient.

"I like being here with my grandsons and daughter, but they eat a lot differently than I do. I'm missing my green vegetable shakes, my shark cartilage, not to mention my ice cream. They won't let me drink my urine!"

"I can do my yoga in the bedroom I share with Mike. He thinks I'm crazy."

"I'm missing out on my meditation and channeling. It's okay. I'll survive ... I hope. Thanks for arranging my care. Most of all I miss your smile."

I miss him, but he's in good hands.

I prayed the best for him and his daughter.

In two weeks I received a call of despair from Betty. "It's not going to work with dad living here. He doesn't like my food, my sons quarreling with each other, or their crazy music. They're teenagers. It seems we fight all the time. Dad's a bachelor and a loner. How can I expect to change him?"

"Besides, I don't want anyone dying in my house. I think it would 'freak out' my boys."

"Would it be possible for dad to return to his place and continue hospice with you?"

"Yes, it's possible. Are you sure this is best?"

I miss the old guy, but not his urine!

"Yes, I'm sure. Please, make those arrangements for dad and especially for me. I'd appreciate it."

Betty drove him back to his home, leaving the red Honda for her son. It was a bitter-sweet pill to swallow for Gary. He was upset because of her rejection, but happy to be independent again.

One transfer consent later, the homing pigeon came back to our hospice. Again, the social worker made the changes to facilitate Gary's return.

In the three weeks Gary spent with his daughter, he had become thinner and weaker. His body had declined, but his spirit to fight his cancer had not wavered.

His had cyanosis in his fingers and toes, and increased shortness of breath. I used my pulse oximeter to check the percentage of oxygen in his blood at rest. It registered eighty-four per cent, an abnormal low. Oxygen therapy was a mandatory for his comfort."

He agreed to stop smoking if I obtained a prescription for Nicorette gum. He began to use his nasal cannula continuously.

"I feel like a new man. I have energy to spare! Maybe I can finish my house now."

Denial is a sanity saver!

He wanted to get his house in order. He ordered a new king size bed, a memory foam mattress, red carpet for his bedroom, a new black dresser for his clothes, and two matching black and red floor lamps. He hung a large black and white picture of Marilyn Monroe above his dresser.

On my visit following the refurnishing of his bedroom, I noticed he could barely get in and out of his new king size bed. He confessed to falling twice. "Oh, I forgot to tell you. You're so busy."

Maybe his brain cancer is altering his decision making process.

A purple bruise on his hip and big bandage on his ankle was a red flag. He was getting weaker with a greater chance to fall and severely injure himself.

Safety first. Soon he will be unable to walk to his bathroom alone. The bathroom is over fifty feet from his bed and in a different part of his house. Who designed this house? Certainly not a woman!

"I'll order you a walker."

"Don't expect me to use it. It's going to end up in the garage. I don't have room for it!"

On my next visit, I found it upside down in the middle of my walkway. I righted it back on its legs and pushed it out of my way!

Can't miss seeing that walker! Four legs straight up! Thankful it's not broken.

After a few more falls and my first aid patch work, Gary consented to using a walker. I brought it in from the garage to help him navigate. I ordered a bed side commode. The equipment company placed it by his bed.

I'm glad I didn't have to put it there. I hope it keeps him from falling.

A week passed and he was extremely short of breath and admitted he could not take a shower. It was time for a home health aide to assist him with his care. He resisted the thought of someone giving him a shower.

"Oh Gary, it might be a lot of fun."

He laughed. "All right, if you'll be here on her first visit to introduce and supervise. Bring your bikini. You might get wet!"

"I might do that." I winked and smiled.

On the first health aide visit, I steadied him as she washed his body in the shower. Gary came out with a big smile on his face. "I think I can get used to this."

I'm right again. He needs a shower bar, not me!

"Gary, to be safe you need a shower bar. I can't be here to hold you every time you shower."

"I'll miss you, but I can only handle one nurse at a time. I guess you're right."

He looked forward to his health aide visit three times a week. She would change his bed linen, give him a massage, and listen to his concerns. She became his confidant.

Unknown to me, a shower bar appeared.

Hope he didn't install it.

Another fall, another injury, this time it was in the bathroom. He couldn't get up. He crawled to his phone and remembered to call hospice. The number was stuck on his phone. When the office contacted me, I called the local fire department on their non-emergency line to assist Gary while I traveled to his home. I arrived after the firemen left. Gary was in his bed with a mischievous grin on his face.

He looks like he swallowed a canary.

"I liked the firegirl! Wouldn't mind if she came every day! Could you arrange that?"

"Keep on falling and they'll keep on coming." I gave him a hug. "She might not always be a she. She might be a he. Sorry, you're stuck with me! I'm always on duty."

I've ordered him a bedside commode so he wouldn't be walking so far to the bathroom. Where is it? I didn't see it in the garage."

"Where is your bedside commode?"

"I had my neighbor put it in the back yard so it wouldn't be in your way. He also installed the shower bar. Doesn't that make you happy?"

"Yes, I'm elated about the bar. I'm disgusted about the bedside commode. You have proved you needed it. I'll go find it and place it here by your bed."

What a mess! The commode was full of dirt and bird poop. After cleaning the commode and placing it by his bed, I got a urinal from my car supplies and gave it to him. "I am ordering you a bedside table to keep this urinal within reach. This commode better be at your bedside when I return on my next visit."

"Oh, I have another gift for you. I'm ordering you a wheelchair so you can roll to your bathroom to take a shower with your personal assistant.

"By the way, did you have a BM today?"

"No, I haven't had one for four days. It's tough to get it out, now-a-days. I use my finger to get it started. Have any suggestions?"

"I can give you an enema."

"Oh no you don't! Any other ideas for a smooth move?"

"I'll increase your routine laxatives. Take two ounces of milk of magnesium tonight. Call me by noon if there is no BM in this bedside commode. I'll come and do the water rotor rooter routine! How's that?"

"That's enough to make me stop meditating and start praying real hard!"

"Great idea!" I laughed. "There is a higher power, you know."

It was obvious the time had come to have a twenty-four hour caregiver. I called the social worker and together we listed Gary's options. His best was locating a previous girlfriend. He called her with his fingers crossed.

"Hi Cindy. It's me."

"I'd know your voice anywhere. How are you?"

85

"Not good. Did I tell you I have lung cancer and it's gone to my brain? It has gotten so bad that I need someone to live with me. It's a lot to ask, but would you be willing to try? I'm unable to walk and I want to die in my own home. I have a wonderful hospice nurse, I love, and she will teach you all you need to know. She has a great sense of humor. Would you like to talk to her?"

"Give me her number and I'll call her after I think about it. I'll call you back.

Cindy called me. After a long conversation she agreed to try her luck at being his hired caregiver.

She called Gary. "Gary? I'll do it, but I'm not a nurse! Remember, I'm your friend."

When Cindy arrived, I was happy to instruct her in simple nursing care and how to administer his medications. Cindy seemed to handle his care and depended on me for emotional support and organizing his meds.

"There's a chart in his folder to help you know when to give him his medications. I've written the names and the times."

"We give some medications only when Gary needs them, not routinely. I've enclosed a yellow pad for you to write the date and times you give these medications."

Cindy was a quick learner and she kept track of every medication she gave.

Even though Gary was cranky and not in control, he realized Cindy was giving him her full support, love, and commitment. This was more than his daughter would do. He decided not to complain or expect instant service.

Since his living situation had changed, I called Betty and informed her about Cindy living with her dad.

"Hello, Betty. This is Karen, with hospice."

"Hi Karen, how are you?"

"I'm okay. Let me give you an update on your dad."

"After many falls, he hired a full time caregiver to live with him. He called one of his former girlfriends, Cindy. She agreed. Do you remember her?"

"Dad has had so many girlfriends, I don't remember any of them, although the name sounds familiar."

"She seems capable and willing to care for him. Your dad is lucky to have her."

"Thanks for keeping me informed. We still are not on talking terms. I wish it were different, but it is the way it is!"

Gary was interested in my conversation with Betty. He was not surprised when he heard that Betty had not offered to help. He was grateful for Cindy.

Gary wanted to reward Cindy, even though he was paying her to care for him. He told me he was going to change his Living Trust and have Cindy be his heir instead of his daughter.

"I know who loves and cares for me at my weakest time in life."

He called his lawyer to meet with him and change his Living Trust and Durable Power Attorney of Health Care. Our social worker and I were there to witness his signature.

Another visit brought another problem. I noticed a big empty orange bucket near his bed.

Strangest thing I've ever seen."

"Gary, tell me about your orange bucket?"

He had a little boy grin on his face. "I like it better than that 'big pot chair' you put beside my bed. That thing you gave me is a bucket under a toilet seat with handles. I had Cindy put it in the garage."

He is hanging on to his autonomy with the big orange bucket. The bucket is rough around the edges and so is he.

I noticed an old white toilet seat alongside the orange bucket. I laughed.

Oh my. That's how you do it? Wow, that's a real yoga balancing act. What if he and the toilet seat slide off the bucket? That would be a catastrophe or a castration!

"Gary, are you sure you won't slide off that orange bucket?"

"Don't worry, I can manage my jewels."

Cindy was standing nearby with her hands on her hips. "Karen, whatcha goin' do? He certainly has some crazy ideas! It seems sadistic."

"Gary, I'm going to find your bedside commode. If you want use your orange bucket you can replace the bedside commode bucket with your bucket. You are not to use your toilet seat on the orange bucket again. You will fall."

The commode was upside down, like the walker, in the garage. It was missing its bucket. I brought it in the house and placed it over the orange bucket. I put his dirty toilet seat in the trash can.

Cindy was holding her sides laughing. "I told you that you would get in trouble with that orange bucket. It scared me every time you sat on it. You were having trouble getting to it, let alone sitting on it. I have to steady you when you're out of bed!"

"Karen, is it possible to get a wheel chair?"

"I already ordered him a wheelchair. It's in the garage."

"That damn wheelchair will stay in the garage with all the rest of your stuff I don't need! I might even paint it red. Does it have a motor?"

"No motor. Would it make a difference?"

"Not to me!"

"If you have the time to paint it, paint it. That's okay with me. But maybe you should paint it orange. It would match your silly old orange poopy bucket! I dare you."

"I might. Can you order me some paint?"

"Sure, why not? The least you can do is use your wheelchair for Cindy's sake no matter what color it is. Think about it Gary."

Soon his daily care became overwhelming. Gary made extra demands on her time. Gary was making Cindy a nervous wreck with his constant haranguing. She was ready to walk out the back door.

I felt her frustrations. It's time to talk with Cindy alone.

"Excuse me Gary, I need some time to talk with Cindy. I'll be right back."

"Cindy, let's go sit on his couch in the living room together."

As we sat down together on the black leather couch, I took Cindy's hand and looked into her eyes. "Tell me how you really feeling."

Tears started to roll down her cheek. "I can't do this. I'm tired. I need help."

"No one can do this job alone." I gave Cindy a big 'K hug.'

A volunteer would be great. She needs 'time out' now!

"Would it help to have a few hours for yourself?"

"I would love a chance to get out of here."

"Maybe you need some additional help. Let me arrange another visit with our social worker."

The social worker came for a visit and suggested a volunteer.

Gary declined. "I'll have my neighbor drop in and she can leave for a few hours if he'll sit with me and talk."

During my next nursing visit, I asked Cindy about the neighbor. "Has the neighbor given you some free time?"

"Gary hasn't even talked to him."

"You and I can talk with the neighbor before I leave today."

The neighbor was willing to sit with Gary for two hours two days a week. Cindy began enjoying four hours a week to relax in town.

Starbucks never tasted better.

Another visit found Cindy and me back on the leather couch. "Karen, he's sleeping more and he is very demanding when he's awake. I can't keep up with his constant ringing of the bell."

"There's a blue booklet in your home folder which tells about the stages Gary will pass through as he gets closer to death. It's called *Gone from my Sight*. When you have a minute you should read it.

Turning towards Cindy, I rested my arm on the back of the couch. I started sharing some changes that would happen in the next few weeks. "Gary is slowly dying. His body will stop working and life will come to an end."

Cindy turned towards me with tears in her eyes as I continued. "Gary is already needing longer periods of sleep as his body functions slow down. He may turn away from you and lay in a fetal position. It would not be unusual for him to 'wake up' and start asking for food or favors. It probably seems to you like a bazaar personality change."

"I've seen him curled up in that fetal position. I wondered why. Now I know."

Taking my arm off the couch and crossing my legs, I placed my elbow on my knee. "Gary's ability to communicate will leave him. He may become confused about the time of day, people's names, and where they live. It will seem like he has lost his memory."

"You will notice a decrease in blood circulation to his skin and limbs. His extremities will be cold to touch. The skin will be bluish purple and blotchy. He may run a fever as he dehydrates."

"As he nears death, Gary will fight to hold onto life, not wanting to let go." I crossed my arms over my heart. "At some point you may need to give him permission to leave."

Cindy reached for my hand. "Will all these things happen?"

"Not all of these changes may happen, but you may experience some of them."

"When he's getting very close to death, he will refuse to eat or drink. His need to urinate will decline. The amount of urine will decrease. He'll need a diaper."

Leaning forward, I placed my other hand on her hand. "As he becomes restless, he might pull at his bed sheets, clothing or pick at the air, which indicates he sees things you cannot see. He will probably need sedation to keep him calm."

"Will you be there to help?"

"Yes, I will be here to show you how to give his medications. It will be necessary to have Gary hire additional help so you can sleep."

"In the active stage of dying, there comes a noisy rattling sound in his breathing. Some refer to it as the 'death rattle.' It is thick mucus and fluid collecting in the throat. He may have periods of rapid breathing or periods when he may not breathe for up to a full minute. His respirations will be irregular and shallow."

"This is a lot for me to remember. I'll read that little blue book."

On the following visit I asked, "Did you have time to read, *Gone from my Sight?*"

"Yes, I did. Now I understand some of the problems I am having with Gary. It seems he is in the early stages of dying, but it's not easy for me. Sometimes I want to wring his neck. There's only relief when he sleeps. He is sleeping a lot more and that's good! Sometimes he can't stop talking, and he's so demanding. I guess it's normal. Thanks for helping me understand. This is all new to me."

"Let me give you a hug." I hugged her tight and could feel the tension leave her body. I whispered, "You can do this. I'm here to help you. I'm a phone call away. Never hesitate to call me, night or day."

Mid November brought cold weather to the desert. Gary's house had no central heating, no dry wall on the inside of the outside walls, and no insulation. His neighbor had given him a portable electric heater, but it was no match for the cold wind which blew through his unfinished two thousand square foot house.

On an unscheduled early morning visit, after the weather turned cold, I found Cindy shivering while wearing two big sweat shirts, three pairs of sweat pants, and a pair of Ug boots with two pairs of long socks. The gas stove in the kitchen had all four burners on high, the oven door was wide open and was set at four hundred degrees.

"You can't have all these burners and the oven on to keep the house warm. You will die of carbon monoxide poisoning." I walked over to the stove and turned off all the burners and the oven.

"You can't take our heat away from us. We'll freeze to death," Cindy complained.

"You must put on more clothing or get in bed with Gary."

I bet he would enjoy snuggling with her again.

"Try and find a coat to wear. Cover Gary with more blankets." I took my pink knitted cap off, walked over to Gary, and placed it on his bald head. "That will keep your head warm. Keep your body under the blankets Cindy puts on you. We'll have a meeting this afternoon to resolve this problem."

"I knew I'd be in trouble if you made an early morning visit. The desert sun eventually warms us up. By the early afternoon we're fine!"

"You look cute in your new pink cap. Think of me while you wear it. I'll be back soon." I kissed him on the cheek. "Good-bye for now, I'll return soon, just like a bad penny!"

This was a critical problem for the social worker and me. When I got in my car, I immediately called her with this problem. That afternoon we met with Gary and Cindy.

The discussion began with the social worker. "We are responsible for the safety of our patients. There are laws in place which require action when a critical safety issue presents itself in the home. Gary, you cannot stay here without heat. We have to find another place. Let's talk about our options."

There aren't too many.

The plan was to place him in a board and care facility licensed for hospice patients. Cindy asked for a place close to her home.

The facility we chose was the Oasis, a residential home owned by a local family. Three other hospice patients were living in the facility. There was one vacant room for Gary.

Winter had not been kind to Gary. He had to leave his home.

We transferred him the next morning by ambulance to the warm Oasis where he was welcomed by the smell of a home cooked meal.

"This won't be so bad. After all, I like the personal care and you'll still be my nurse." Gary was unable to walk so he ate his small meals in bed. He spent the day watching TV or listening to music. He had a private quiet room, perfect for his meditation.

Peace and quiet is medicine for the soul.

Cindy brought his shaving kit, clothes, personal items, and a framed picture of them skiing.

She looked at me and laughed. "Darn, I forgot his old orange bucket!"

"He doesn't need it. He can't stand alone and bear his own weight. He's bed bound. He has to use his urinal with the assistance of the staff."

I called Betty with the change in his living quarters. "I was expecting your call. I knew the house would never be warm enough in winter. How's he doing?"

"He's lost more weight and is unable to stand alone, but he's still his old feisty self."

"Thank you for taking care of him. He burned his bridges when he called me and told me he was taking me off his will. We're not on speaking terms. I don't know what's going to happen to him. He has such strange ideas about life and death." I listened and my heart ached as she talked about eternity.

"I have tried my best to please my dad all my life, but it has never worked. I'm not sure a visit at this time would change anything. Besides, I can't bear to see him. I'd rather keep the memory of his surprise visit, when he gave Mike the old red Honda. By the way, tell him it runs like a charm."

"Hopefully he knows I love him. Would you please tell him I love him for being my dad?"

"Yes, I'll tell him." I told Gary his daughter's message. He cried.

His daughter never visited him at the Oasis.

Eventually Gary graduated from bed pan to diapers.

He would smile on my visits when I teased him about his old orange bucket.

"Guess what?"

"What?"

"Cindy took the old orange bucket and planted flowers in it. They seem to grow very well!"

He grinned. "At least I had a seat on my bucket. I bet no one else can brag about that!"

Gary's home health aide continued to provide emotional support and hygiene care. The chaplain gave Gary spiritual support and prayer.

Gary believed he would move on to a higher level of consciousness. His consciousness would continue after death and be in a different form, like a spirit. He had told me about his spirit going to a different planet. He equated his higher power as one with the universe. "Maybe God will find a way to reincarnate me somewhere. I hope it's not a jack-rabbit!"

When Cindy visited him, she sat by him for hours holding his hand. The silence between them was golden and there were no words to explain how they felt.

After a week, Cindy called in tears. "How can Gary continue like this? He barely recognizes me. He can't talk anymore. It must be horrible for him."

"Cindy, Gary's spirit is ready but his heart is strong. When it's the right time, his spirit will leave his body."

"Maybe he will land on Venus. That's what he tells me. When I look at the night sky and see Venus, I'll be seeing him."

Gary lived only three weeks at the Oasis. He died two days before Christmas.

The Oasis' staff called and informed me of a change in his breathing pattern. They requested I come immediately and be with him.

When I arrived, he was drenched in perspiration and extremely short of breath. I gave him medication to help him breathe easier and relax. It worked. I called Cindy hoping she could see Gary one more time.

"Gary, It is okay to let go. You've fought this fight long enough." He could not fully open his eyes or speak. "I'm right here beside you. I'll not leave you. I've called Cindy and she is coming."

He lightly squeezed my hand. I knew he could hear me. I started singing his favorite Christmas carol, *Silent Night*.

Silent Night,
Holy Night,
All is calm,
All is bright.
'Round yon virgin,
Mother and Child,
Holy Infant,
So tender and mild,
Sleep in heavenly peace ...

As I sang that phrase, he released my hand, took a quick short gasp, and his spirit left.

... Sleep in heavenly peace.

I cried, so grateful to be with him when his angel took him. Cindy had not made it in time.

With his last breath, his body was at peace but his eyes needed closing. I closed his eyelids and took a moment to pray Gary's memory would live on with his daughter, grandsons and girlfriend.

After gently washing his face and body for the last time, I took a moment to remember the challenging times with Gary.

It was time to gather Gary's narcotics and other medications. I sat with the staff by his bedside. We counted and discarded the meds according to their protocol.

After charting his final visit, I waited for Cindy to arrive. She came through the door with her tear stained face.

"Cindy, I am so sorry for your loss. He died ten minutes ago."

"I was hoping I would have been here when he passed."

"I'm glad you're here now. You were his earth angel. How are you?"

"I'm okay, I guess. I'm thankful you were with him." She hugged me tight. "You were a wonderful nurse."

"Thank you, Cindy."

"Tell me about his final moments."

"While I was singing *Silent Night*, he left us. I heard him take his last breath. It seemed the right song to sing before Gary took flight. It's only two days before Christmas."

Cindy wanted time alone with him. I left the room and phoned Betty, his doctor, the hospice team, his pharmacy, the equipment company, and lastly his mortician.

When Cindy came from his room, she said, "He's finally at rest. Thank you for being with him when he died."

"Do you need more time with Gary?"

"No, Gary's wishes were to be cremated. The mortuary will contact me for his ashes. Every night I'll look for him in the sky and find him in my thoughts forever."

She gave me a big hug, turned, and walked out of the Oasis.

Gary was a warrior. He had fought the brave battle against the dragon of cancer. He had tried everything he knew to stop its rage. Only when he accepted the finality of his cancer was he able to face death with peace.

"By which the rising sun will come to us from heaven to shine on those living in darkness and in the shadow of death, to guide our feet into the paths of peace."
Luke 1:78, 79 (NIV)

THE LONG WAIT
Howard Ellowis
(2004)

He is long gone, but the thought of him remains,

Today my father was roused from a corner of my mind.

It seemed time for this meeting to take place,

We have been strangers for many years,

His death did not separate us,

That happened while he was still alive.

I remember being called home from work.

I arrived to find him lifeless in the sun room.

There was no shock or grief at seeing him dead,

I feared him in life, I feared him in death.

His gift to me, a product of his daily rage.

Now I reclaim the memory of my father,

I want to give it a new setting in my mind,

I want to come home again and cry this time,

I want to say now that we are not so different,

I want to love him now.

I have lived the difficulties of life,

I can match his rage and frustrations,

They are familiar to me now . . .

I see both of us as frail.

I give this gift to both of us,

The waiting enhances its sweetness,

**(From *The Long Wait* by Howard Ellowis,
used by permission)**

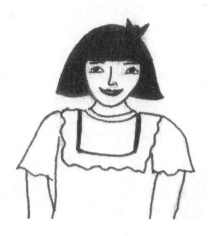

I FOUND MY LOST DAUGHTER!

Church was over and my husband and I were heading to the parking lot. "Hey, Karen, we'd like to go to lunch with you. Do you have the time?"

It was Ella. Ella lived in my neighborhood and we spent time playing Mexican train dominoes with her parents. "Sure, we'd love it. How about Rosa's Cantina?"

"Meet you there in five."

It was our local hangout. It was usually busy after church on Sunday. We said hello to several of our friends as we settled into a red Naugahyde padded wood booth. Ella and Matt arrived at the same time as our menus. I ordered a taco salad while my husband had a taco and chili relleno plate. Ella and Matt shared a sizzling fajita plate.

Nothing like the taste of Mexico!

As we started to enjoy the meal, Ella asked me, "How can you work with the dying? Isn't that depressing to you?"

"Not at all. I look at dying differently than most people. Everyone will die, guaranteed. Dying is the process required for our spirit to leave the body. The spirit longs to be set free. To me, death is our final victory."

"The Bible says it best: 'Death has been swallowed up in victory. Where, O death, is your victory? Where, O death, is your sting?'" (1 Corinthians 15:54, 55) (NIV).

"Hospice allows the patient and family a multifaceted support system. This includes emotional, spiritual, pain and symptom management, medication, medical equipment, and hygiene care. It provides the opportunity for a patient to die well. It is a privilege to share the last chapter of life with them."

"I can only imagine the positive energy you give to your patients. It must be a joy to have you as a nurse."

"Well, that's a compliment bigger than I deserve. Thank you."

"Bottom line is I have an uncle who needs your love and care. I would like to see him on hospice and have you as his nurse."

"Tell me more about him."

"Uncle Stan lives alone. His doctor recently diagnosed him with terminal pancreatic cancer. His wife died on hospice two years ago. I'm sure he will be going onto hospice soon. He's so weak, he can no longer drive his old Chevy pickup to the store. He's in horrible pain and so nauseated he can't eat solid food. Seven Up is his main source of energy."

"Is he still walking?"

"He walks slowly with a walker around in his mobile home and complains of continuous pain throughout his entire body. He looks like a walking skeleton and has lost his motivation to live. It's so sad."

"Does he have family to help him?"

"My husband and I realize how busy his family is with their children. They don't have the time or room to help him. We're retired and would be willing to have him live with us during his final days. If we had him come to live with us, would it be possible to have you as his nurse."

"Since you're in my neighborhood, I would be the nurse assigned to him. Have his doctor call my hospice office and fax an order for his admission. Here's my business card with all the information you'll need. I think I've met Uncle Stan. I'd be honored to be his nurse."

"Karen, I've never had a child to nurture and maybe this is my chance to take care of someone who needs me."

The care of her critically ill uncle will not be an easy job, but helping him through dying would be an experience she will never forget and never regret.

The conversation turned to politics and vacations. The meal satisfied our Mexican cravings. The chips and salsa never ended until we said uncle!

No room for dessert and I love flan.

Ella decided to call Uncle Stan and take him to his next doctor visit. The doctor acknowledged Stan's life would soon end. Uncle Stan requested my hospice. The doctor honored his request.

Often the doctor chooses the hospice he prefers without consulting the patient. Uncle Stan is exercising his choice. Good for him.

The following morning Stan's doctor faxed the order to start hospice. My nursing supervisor assigned me as his case manager. Uncle Stan would be living in Ella's home.

Ella and Matt prepared a room for Uncle Stan in their newly built home. He moved into their guest bedroom with white wooden shutters and white framed nature scenes on three walls.

When Uncle Stan entered his bright yellow room, he was surprised to see a hospital bed with an alternating air pressure mattress.

"Ella, I'll miss my queen size bed. Couldn't we have brought it from my mobile home? It would be a lot more comfortable."

Ella seemed puzzled. "Your queen size bed will barely fit in this room. It will be very hard to help you in that large

103

bed in this small room. Maybe you can get comfortable in this bed."

"Let me try." His walker taxied him to the bed and he sat down. He stretched his body onto the air mattress. Ella took the remote and brought his body up to a sitting position.

"Does you bed allow you to sit up like this?"

"No, on second thought, this bed might help me breathe easier and give me a better night's sleep. You sold me, if I can keep the bed rails down."

"It's kind of you and Matt to care for me in your home. The least I can do is be happy with this hospital bed. If it will help you care for me, I'm all for it."

Ella reached into his suit case. "Let me help you put these pictures of your wife and children on the dresser. That will make you feel a little more at home."

Ella phoned me and told me Uncle Stan had moved in and was expecting a visit. "I can be there tomorrow. Is ten o'clock okay?"

"Perfect. I can't wait to see you."

"Thanks, I'll be there."

Ella was waiting for me at her beautifully etched glass door. Uncle Stan heard me as I walked on the stone tiled hallway. "Hi Karen, Ella told me you'll be my nurse. It's hard to believe. Please call me Uncle Stan. I'll call you Nurse Karen." I agreed as he winked at me with the cutest smile.

Uncle Stan sat on the soft suede couch hugging a multicolored cotton quilt. "This is a gift from Ella who hand stitched it for me. She knows I'm always cold."

Ella reached over and wrapped the quilt tightly around him like a baby.

Maybe he is her baby. Lucky for Uncle Stan!

Explaining the hospice benefit funded by Medicare was easy since he had been his wife's primary caregiver. Most of the questions came from Ella and Matt. Uncle Stan was happy to sign the hospice consents for admission. He knew it was inevitable.

"Do not call nine-one-one in an emergency or at the time of death. Please call the hospice number any time for problems or questions."

Uncle Stan shared his medical history. "My doctor made it clear to me I will not be here for Easter and it's only three months away. I'll really miss the ham dinner with my family, but my new body won't need food," as he pointed to the ceiling. "For sure, I won't be nauseated or in pain."

"I am nauseated from my cancer. It makes it difficult for me to eat. Almost everything that goes down comes up. Vomiting and pain are the worst. Is there was a way to stop them? I have completed all my cancer treatments and do not want to go back to the hospital under any circumstances!"

"I want to live comfortably until I die, if it is possible."

"I'll call your doctor and get medication to control your pain and vomiting. The pharmacy will deliver it to your door later today. I'll call Ella and give her instructions on how to administer it. How does that sound?"

"Sounds good to me."

Uncle Stan turned to Ella. "I am happy to be in your home, but I feel guilty intruding on your privacy. I know it's hard."

"Uncle Stan, we're happy to have you stay with us. You'll not be a burden."

"I'm glad to hear that. I know living here will keep me from interrupting my boys' busy lives. Maybe they'll come visit me."

"Uncle Stan. Here is your hospice folder. What do you remember about hospice?"

"It was a big help to me during those difficult times caring for my wife. I appreciated the help of the nurses and especially the home health aides. They took good care of Florence."

"Would twice a week for the health aide be sufficient?"

"Yes, that would be good."

"Would you like a chaplain?"

"Sure. If he is in the area, please have him stop by."

"A medical social worker's visit is mandatory. I will have him call and set up a time? Ella, you may have some questions he can address."

"This is new to us taking care of someone very sick. All we have ever taken care of is our dog, Cookie."

"Ella, do you think you and Matt may need time together away from the house? Would a volunteer be of help to you?"

"Yes. I would love to have a date night with Matt. How often can a volunteer come?"

"That's between you and your volunteer. I'll contact our volunteer coordinator and she'll call you."

"Uncle Stan, would a wheelchair be helpful?"

"Is it small enough to put in Ella's trunk? I would love to attend church."

"Yes. I'll order you a light weight wheelchair and you should get it tomorrow."

"I'm a lucky man to have you as my nurse."

Having you as a patient is a blessing to me.

"When is your next visit?"

"I'll see you on Friday. That's in two days."

Twice a week I started my day sharing a fresh cup of coffee as we visited in the living room. We sang his favorite Gospel songs. He told me he enjoyed listening to his Gospel Music DVD's every day. He had all the words memorized.

It became routine to listen to his lung and heart sounds, take his blood pressure, and check his skin for changes. I would ask him about his level of pain and nausea. "It's not perfect, but it's a lot better."

His pancreatic cancer made it mandatory to continually increase the dosage for his insurmountable pain. At every visit I would call his doctor to give an update on his status.

The black and white cocker spaniel, Cookie, was great company for him. He taught the dog new tricks. I often found Uncle Stan holding Cookie on his lap feeding him doggie treats.

No wonder he got that name!

He would give me a dog cookie and tell me, "You never know when you may need this in your travels. Maybe it will help keep you safe from a dog bite!"

It's true. You never know when a dog will bite. I had a dog bite me in the face when I was four!

In our conversations, I would listen to his feelings. He would tell me how difficult it was to fall asleep. I would inform his doctor of his insomnia and obtain orders for his anxiety.

He always wanted to pray for me at the end of each visit. I guess he knew I needed it.

Uncle Stan had a chart in his hospice folder listing all updated medications. In this folder the nurse and other hospice team members charted their visits and pertinent changes.

This is a great resource for team communication.

When Uncle Stan became too short of breath to sing and talk in full sentences, I ordered him a home oxygen concentrator and four portable tanks in case there was a power failure. It improved his singing and his spirit.

Amazing what a little oxygen can do.

One day Uncle Stan had a very important request. He wanted to see his daughter he never knew from birth. His girlfriend conceived her prior to his tour of duty in Korea. He only found out about her birth when he returned home. By then his girlfriend had married someone else. She did not want him to visit or be in their daughter's life.

He only remembered his missing daughter's full maiden name and in what state she lived thirty-five years ago. I conferred with the hospice medical social worker. He accepted the challenge and started a search on the internet. Julie's information eventually popped up on the screen.

Our social worker was excited and stopped me in the hallway. "I found the Stan's missing daughter. How soon can I let him know?"

"As soon as possible!"

Being excited is an understatement. This makes my day. No, it makes my whole year!

The social worker arranged a co-visit. "Stan, I have good news. I have found your missing daughter! I have her married name, telephone, and address. How do you feel about talking to her?"

"Scared to death! Don't even know if she wants to see me. Now what do I do?"

"You could have Ella call her? She could be a buffer. How does it sound to you?"

"That sounds good."

"Karen, could you share this with Ella? Would you coach her on what to say?"

"I'll do that."

Before we left the house, I met with Ella and made a few suggestions for the conversation including Stan's willingness to pay for her flight.

When Ella called, Julie could not believe her father had found her and she wanted to meet him.

"Julie, you're invited to come and stay at our home with your dad. You can come and stay as long as you want. Uncle Stan's happy to pay for your round trip ticket from Pennsylvania."

The big question is, will she come?

Julie had always wondered where her father lived and if she looked like him. Most of all she wanted to know if she could love him and he could love her after all these years. She decided to accept her dad's offer and took a plane from Pennsylvania.

The family enjoyed a celebration where she met her five step-brothers for the first time. She was able to forgive her dad, resolve her personal issues, and begin a short and sweet relationship.

Our hospice social worker saved the day again. They are experts in issues of the heart!

After Julie returned home, she made it a habit to call her dad every Saturday and Wednesday. Uncle Stan would always ask, "What day is it? Is it Saturday or Wednesday yet?"

Uncle Stan soon became too weak to walk. He could not bear his own weight and only with assistance could he transfer to the bedside commode for his 'daily duty,' as Matt called it. Ella was unable to do physical lifting due to her injured back. Her strong retired husband did all the lifting and turning. Uncle Stan only weighed one hundred pounds soaking wet. He had lost sixty-five pounds during his short illness.

Lying in bed was becoming a real drag. He did not like his hospital bed, but he admitted the rails helped him when he wanted to move, especially when he needed to reposition himself to the top of the bed.

Complete bed rest has complications. I taught him to do bed aerobics to increase his circulation and prevent blood clots from forming in his lower legs. He faithfully rotated his ankles by making foot circles, stretched his feet up and down, and splayed his fingers and toes during every TV commercial.

On each visit I would always ask him, "Did you do your 'bed aerobics' today?"

He would give me that little wrinkled smile and say, "Sure did, I tried my best."

He loved ice cream, especially Ben and Jerry's. His favorite was chocolate marble. His ice cream habit came in handy when he could no longer swallow his pills. Ella would crush them in a coffee grinder and mix them in his ice cream. It worked like a charm. He never knew he was taking medicine.

It's a happy habit not all caregivers know about.

Days seemed like weeks, and weeks seemed like months for Stan. He wanted this struggle to end. He was learning the body fights hard to stay alive. He would ask at each visit, "How long will it be? What's your best guess? Why does it take so long?"

"The answer is always the same. It will be at the right time."

Maybe God hasn't completed your heavenly house or maybe He's waiting for one more prayer.

He was very appreciative of all the tender care Ella gave. He only wished he could pay her back in a tangible way. I reminded him, "Matt and Ella were once rookies, but because of you, they are super star caregivers."

"Ella might be, but not Matt."

Matt had a great sense of humor. Nothing was ever serious. He and Uncle Stan would tease each other. One day Matt made a cookie filled with prunes for Uncle Stan and told him it was a chocolate chip cookie. Uncle Stan's gustatory cells (taste buds) and olfactory cells (smell buds) were diminishing and he never realized there were prunes in the cookie! Matt discovered his uncle was 'moved' by his soft cookie when he emptied the bucket of his bedside commode!

Weeks later Uncle Stan was unable to transfer to the commode and he began wearing diapers. Ella enlisted Matt to change his diaper. After his first diaper change, Matt made a game of diapering by using a purple hand towel to cover his privates and one liner jokes.

There is never a dull moment in this house.

Ella confided with me, "Julie calls every Saturday and Wednesday to talk with her dad. She tells me, 'I want to hear his voice one more time and tell him I love him.'"

In addition to calls to her dad, she called me for updates on his condition. At the end of my report I would tell her, "Your dad talks about you during each visit. He was grateful

110

he was able to see you and to tell you how sorry he is for not being a part of your life. He loves you very much."

Uncle Stan wanted to write a letter to Julie but he was too weak to hold a pen. He dictated this letter and I mailed it to her.

Dear Julie,

Thank you for visiting me. I know it was a very difficult decision and it turned out wonderful for me. You showed your love by coming and spending a week.

I did not tell you my secret while you were here. I have carried a picture of you as a baby in my wallet ever since your mother sent it to me. It was the only memory I had of you. You were beautiful as a baby and you are even more beautiful as a grown woman.

Not only are you beautiful to my eyes, you are beautiful to my heart. Thank you for being so loving and understanding.

I am proud to be your dad. I am proud of your accomplishments.

I was praying my whole life I would be able to see you and tell you how sorry I was for not being in your life. I was always hoping I could find you. I did not know how. I kept you in my heart and in my prayers.

Our heavenly Father heard my prayers and brought us together.

Your phone calls are a blessing to me. I know I will not ever see you again on this earth, but I look forward to greeting you as you arrive at heaven's gate.

I love you and look forward to seeing you again. May God bless you always.

Love and prayers,
Your Dad

To accompany this letter, I enclosed a picture of Stan holding her hand.

She later shared the letter and photo were keepsakes from her dad's heart and she will treasure them always.

I am sure she is grateful for that memory of spending time with her dad. They do look alike. Maybe it's in their facial expressions, certainly not their hair!

Uncle Stan loved to hear me read the Bible. As it neared Easter Sunday he asked me to read John chapter eleven. Verse twenty-five was his favorite. Jesus said, "I am the resurrection and the life. He who believes in me will live, even though he dies. Whoever lives and believes in me will never die." Easter meant eternal life for Uncle Stan.

"When I was fifty-two, a friend told me that faith in Jesus would change my life forever. I found that faith when I admitted my sin to God, believed Jesus Christ had died to pay the penalty for my sin, and asked Him to be my Savior and Lord. I found this truth after a life of rebellion and alcohol. I call this a mystery miracle. Christ lives in me, the hope of eternal life in glory."

"Karen, I wonder what my heavenly body will look like. Will I recognize my grandma who spoke of this same faith?"

"What do you think?"

"When Christ came back from the grave He had a body that was identified by his disciples. It seems to me that we will have recognizable bodies in heaven if they are like Christ's resurrected body."

"I think you're right."

Stan's earthly body became too weak to sing. He was transitioning in his mind from this earthly life to his new life. He asked me to sing an old Gospel song, *I Can't Feel at Home in this World Any More.* Each time I sang it, he would hold my hand and shed tears.

Sometimes it was difficult to finish the song. When this happened, we would hold hands, cry, and pray silently.

These are tears of inner peace, not sadness without hope.

The week before Uncle Stan died, he could no longer swallow his melted chocolate marble ice cream or suck on a slice of watermelon for fluid. His mouth and lips became very dry and he was only able to mouth his words. I remember him mouthing to me, "I think I could spit cotton, I'm so dry!"

Ella would sit tirelessly beside him and offer him a tiny chip of ice to melt on his tongue. She used water and a special pink mint tasting sponge swab to clean his mouth and teeth. She covered his lips with lip balm.

Ella and Matt would carefully turn Uncle Stan every two hours and reposition his legs with pillows to keep him comfortable. He could no longer thank them, but he could smile.

It became too difficult for Matt and Ella to care for him twenty-four hours a day. They decided to hire someone to help them through the night hours.

Soon he could no longer swallow his pills. There was not a duragesic patch large enough to equal his oral pain medication. It was necessary to continue his pain medication by the use of a sub-cutaneous needle regulated by a controlled administering device (CAD) pump. Matt gave him rectal suppositories for his vomiting every six hours.

His heart rate increased, while his blood pressure decreased. He was breathing rapidly and taking shallow breaths through his mouth. I changed his oxygen from a nasal cannula to a face mask and increased the flow to four liters per minute. It helped him stay comfortable.

Uncle Stan's kidneys continued to close down. I told Matt and Ella he would slowly stop urinating and become more agitated and confused. "I think Uncle Stan will leave us within the next few days."

He died holding Ella's hand early in the morning three days before Easter.

Ella called. "He's gone. Can you come?"

"I'll be there in forty minutes."

"That's okay. I'll call his sons. They will need time to get here."

When I arrived I found Matt, Ella, and his sons sitting at Stan's bedside. He was lying flat on his back with Cookie curled up in a little ball at his feet. It seemed like Cookie knew something was different.

He was finally at peace. I bent over his lifeless body, placed my hand on his heart. It was quiet. With my eyes filled with tears and a lump in my throat, I could barely speak.

"He's home. He's in heaven without pain enjoying his new transformed body."

I'm sure he rode on the wings of angels to his final home. What a ride!

Ella folded her hands together. "He missed celebrating Jesus Christ's resurrection with us, but he made it in time to celebrate in heaven with his Lord and beloved wife."

Matt put his arms around his wife. "Uncle Stan has passed through the storm of death to a safe harbor."

The son holding his father's hand look at me. "Dad was a man of faith in God. He believed in the death and resurrection of Jesus Christ. He wasn't afraid to die. He had peace with his maker."

Nodding my head in agreement, I smiled. "He must be dancing with the angels. I bet he's dancing to his favorite Gospel music! Do you want to hear the music he listened to every day?"

His sons looked at each other. "Yes, that would be great."

I turned on Uncle Stan's DVD player for the last time.

Let the music begin. Music will begin the healing of their grieving hearts. There's something special about music that speaks to the soul of our emotions.

As the music filled the room, I led Ella and Matt to the kitchen. It gave his sons time to be alone with their dad. It gave me an opportunity to thank Ella and Matt for their selfless love and special care they gave to Uncle Stan.

Ella put her arms out to embrace me. "Ella, Uncle Stan was a fortunate man to have a niece like you and an 'almost son' like Matt. You both took time to usher him into his eternal home with dignity and love. What more could he have asked for? Thank you from Uncle Stan."

I made several telephone calls: the hospice team, his doctor, the pharmacy, the equipment company, and the mortuary.

While we were waiting for the mortuary's transportation, I listened as Matt and Ella called Julie. When they handed me the phone, she thanked me. "I will never forget the kindness I felt when I was with you, Ella, Matt, dad, and my brothers. Thanks to dad, I have five new wonderful brothers. I will miss him." I listened to her grateful heart as she cried.

We waited together until the mortuary's white van drove onto the driveway. A professionally dressed man and woman stepped from the van and introduced themselves to the family and gave their condolences.

Removing Uncle Stan's body was very difficult for his sons. They asked for more time alone with their dad.

After the sons said their final good-byes, the attendants wrapped his body in a white sheet and gently lifted his lifeless form to the gurney. His sons chose to walk beside their dad to the vehicle and watch his body leave.

I believe this is the hardest moment of all ... it's final.

As the van eased down the driveway, I listened to their tears.

They thanked Matt and Ella for their care. Each son thanked me with a big hug.

Five hugs of gratitude! No wonder I love being a hospice nurse!

I ended the visit by counting his remaining narcotics with Ella cosigning that we had discarded them properly in a Zip Lock bag of kitty litter. I discarded them in their trash bin.

In my last conversation with Ella, I told her what I remembered most about Uncle Stan. "I remember the smile on his face when he saw his daughter and the enjoyment of his gospel music."

Uncle Stan had found the resolution of a lifelong quest and his reason for living. His strong faith quenched his fear of dying.

He understood the warmth of Ella's colorful quilt. It was always on his bed. Did it make him secure? I think it did. It must have been a feeling of his family's love around him. Hospice helped him place the last piece in his life's quilt.

Thank you hospice team for being that human quilt of many shapes and colors, when sown together, gave Uncle Stan love, hope, and dignity through his storm of dying. We were like an anchor, holding him safe in his turbulent storm.

Uncle Stan may not have remembered all you said or did, but he knew how you made him feel. Stay at it.

All things work together for good for those who love the
Lord …Romans 8:28 (KJV)

FEAR
Marge Anselma
2015

Lord Jesus, I need You to hold my hand,

to comfort me, and tell me You Understand

just how I feel. I'm in such distress.

God, I can't handle this awful mess.

I give it all to You. Take it from me

as you took my sins, when on that tree.

You suffered more than words can tell,

and Lord, 'though I'm afraid, I know full well,

that You will undertake and work things out.

I know in my heart beyond a doubt

that You love me with a love beyond compare,

And will not let me suffer more than I can bear.

Lord Jesus, how thankful I am to know

that You understand, because you suffered so.

Forgive me, Lord, that I have such fear.

I know I can trust You. You're always there.

Just waiting for me to call upon the Name

of the One who always stays the same.

Dear God, I love You so very much.

I need the warmth of Your gentle touch.

Help me to know when the going gets rough

that the grace You supply is always enough.

O, thank You, Father, for You love me so

that I needn't ever fear, because you'll never

let me go.

(Used by permission of the author)

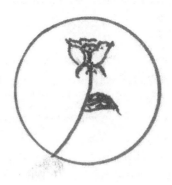

WHERE'S ERNIE?

The yummy smell of fresh bread baking filled my nostrils with memories of days gone by when I entered the front door of the Rose Garden nursing facility.

The aroma takes me back to the infamous bread machine that kneaded the dough, caused it to rise, and even baked my bread. I am sure that is why I lost my girlish figure, when I baked homemade bread for my family every week in one of those bread machines!

Arriving at the front desk to sign the Rose Garden visitor's register, I asked the lobby receptionist, "Where is the fresh bread? It's only ten in the morning and it smells like it's time for lunch."

The young attractive receptionist stared at my badge, gave me a great big smile, and said, "Back again Karen? You should know the smell of fresh bread covers a multitude of odors. I have never seen or tasted that phantom bread, and I've worked here for five years!"

"I'm on a mission today to find Ernie," I told her. "Do you know where I can find him?"

"He could be anywhere," she replied. "Why don't you ask one of the nurses?"

Over fifty patients diagnosed with Alzheimer's disease lived within these walls.

It was my assignment to find Ernie, a patient diagnosed with end stage Alzheimer's disease. He was here, somewhere! I walked to the nursing station and asked the charge nurse, "Where's Ernie?"

"You will find him behind the double doors that are locked at the end of the hall. To unlock the doors push in the numbers 2-2-4-6 and the doors will open to a three ring circus. Be careful none of them escape!"

As I glanced in the rooms along the hall, I remembered the agony of growing old in an extended care facility. I saw a confused patient trying to fit a pair of socks on his hands. In another room, there was an elderly female patient stark naked lying face down on her twin bed without a pillow. She was rubbing a blanket close to her lips. An elderly man was standing at his doorway, loudly pointing at me uncomprehendingly crying words. I thought he was warning me of impending danger when he said repeatedly, "I'm locked in here. They locked me in. They locked me in. Get me out."

Further down the hall sat an elderly woman in her wheelchair caressing a baby doll in her arms singing the words, "Lullaby and good-night" over and over again. Coming towards me was a bright red-haired woman yelling, "I'm dying! I'm dying! I'm dying!" It seemed like those were the only words she could say.

My heart breaks for these confused and fragile patients.

The facility staff, assisting the patients, looked frazzled and tired of trying to do the impossible, keeping everyone safe and comfortable. One seemed to be looking at me to give her a minute to help lift or turn a patient. I paused in the hallway and decided to help her.

It only takes a minute to be kind.

As I came to the locked double doors, I pushed in the secret number code and heard the latch click. The door opened slowly towards me. Holding my arms out wide and motioning for everyone to step back into the room, I started singing to them, "Row, row, row your boat..." The surprised patients backed away and started singing and rowing with me! I looked around the room. Along the walls were flowered couches, old chairs, several stained upholstered chairs, and recliners that could not recline. In the center was a big circular table where many residents were doing crafts and blowing up balloons.

Some were yelling. Others were watching TV half asleep. A few were wearing big colorful bibs while leaning or drooling on each other's shoulders. The staff was feeding the remaining patients snacks of yogurt as it drooled down their chins.

In a loud voice I said, "Where's Ernie? Is he in this room?"

A staff member, who was trying to read with a few patients, said, "He's down at the end of the hall. It's a locked room where he lives with his wife. Their daughter's already in the room waiting for you. Knock on the door. If they don't answer, I have the key. Oh, it's room thirty-eight."

Room thirty-eight's green door had a one-way peep hole at eye level surrounded by a wreath of purple and yellow flowers. They could see me but I could not see them. I knocked loudly on the door.

An attractive brunette opened the door. "Hi, you must be Karen. I'm Debbie. We're expecting you. Please come in. This is my dad, Ernie, and mom, Thelma."

There sat Ernie and Thelma rocking comfortably in their worn chairs of brown and black imitation leather. Debbie was trying to tell them about hospice and appeared stressed, ready for a good glass of wine!

I sat down on the end of their soft squeaky double bed. "Hi, I'm Karen. What's your name?"

Ernie looks fragile and is entering the final stage of Alzheimer's. It certainly is the disease of the brain that breaks the family's heart.

Ernie continued to rock and did not answer my question.

The lights are on but nobody's home.

I gently put my hand on his knee and waited for him to stop rocking. "Are you Ernie?" He shook his head as he looked away from me.

Since I had spent fifteen minutes reading Ernie's medical H & P (History and Physical) at the office, I knew Ernie's past medical condition.

End stage kidney failure is the underlying condition for his prognosis of six months.

The doctor had diagnosed him with Alzheimer's nine years prior.

Taking Debbie's hand I began the conversation. "How long has you dad lived here?"

He is seventy-six years old and he looks ninety.

"About two years. Mom joined him a year ago."

"Hospice will not extend or shorten Ernie's life. We will try and help him through his final days with comfort and dignity."

Debbie gave me a slight smile and began to shake her head. "Looking at dad, you would never believe he built every wall you see around this facility. That was when he was forty years old. He loved working with his hands creating beautiful things of stone and mortar. Before dad knew he had Alzheimer's, he designed the rose garden that is located right behind the patio. He also planted twenty different rose bushes among the angels that he placed in the garden."

She stared into my eyes with tears. "Dad didn't want to end up with this disease. His dad died from vascular dementia, probably Alzheimer's, at eighty-four in a veteran's hospital in New York. His identical twin brother died in this facility two years ago with a stroke, before dad was admitted."

"I realize you're here today because dad has about six months to live. I'm not sure dad understands, but I've talked with his doctor and I do. I'm his voice. I have his medical power of attorney. Do you need it?"

"Is it in his chart at the nurse's station?"

"Yes, they've copied of it."

"Then I have it."

Debbie was realistic concerning her father's prognosis. "I have watched him lose sixty pounds and become more childlike in his behavior over the past four years."

Ernie has mobility problems, limited cognitive abilities, hypertension, and chronic kidney failure with an indwelling Foley catheter.

"It was dad's construction company that provided for our family. There were six children.

"Six children? Where do they live?

"All three of my sisters and both of my brothers live out of state on the east coast. They only see mom and dad once a year, if that often."

"Will they be involved in his care?"

"No. It's not they don't care about them, but it's they live so far away. They're busy with their own jobs and children. Dad has thirteen grandchildren and many great grandchildren."

"I will be the one responsible for his care. Keep in touch with me. I'll keep my family informed."

I sensed the weight of the world on Debbie's shoulders. "Do you know what hospice means?"

"No, not really. But I'd like you to tell me about it and how you think hospice can help dad." After a question and answer discussion explaining hospice, Debbie smiled and said, "I never knew there were so many different occupations that would help the elderly at the end of their lives. I think this is what dad needs now. I feel a lot better already knowing you will be here to help."

She thought a hospice volunteer to visit her parents every week would be helpful. She told me her dad probably would not want a hospice chaplain because he never went to church while raising them.

"I guess he never wanted to take valuable time away from his family on Sunday. It was his day of rest. He was raised Catholic. Maybe a visit from a priest would be helpful."

I agreed to ask our hospice chaplain to contact a priest and give his name to Debbie.

Debbie thought her dad could benefit from extra hygiene care given by the hospice home health aide twice a week. She decided she would like the hospice medical social worker to meet with her so they could discuss any financial assistance available. Her parents' Social Security checks were paying the nursing facility charges, but she was paying for Ensure, co-payments for medications, and diapers.

Debbie asked if hospice could help her make the funeral arrangements for Ernie. I gave her a hug and told her our social worker would visit and help her with those decisions.

"Debbie, I will be making two nursing visits a week to check Ernie's blood pressure, lungs, edema, and care. I promise to call you for any medication changes we would need to keep him comfortable and safe. You can call me any time for concerns or questions that may arise."

Debbie stayed with her parents while I left to talk with the charge nurse.

After talking with her, I scanned the facility's chart to check all the present orders. I copied all of Ernie's medications onto our hospice medication profile. I made a list of medications for which hospice would be financially responsible. Then I notified the hospice team and Ernie's doctor regarding his admission. Ernie's referring doctor would be responsible for new orders. The hospice doctor would be on call twenty-four hours a day to oversee his palliative/end of life care.

In the conference room, I gave Debbie a list of medications her father was taking. I identified which medications hospice would cover by placing a star next to each one. Hospice would pay for only those related to his disease diagnosis that qualified him. It also would cover all comfort medications.

Ending this conversation I asked her, "Do you feel comfortable to make this decision for your dad?"

Her words were slow, realizing this was the last step in her dad's journey of life. "Yes, I think dad is ready for hospice."

"I can't believe you won't charge us. I wish dad could understand how helpful it will be for him and me."

"I'm in agreement at the time of death there will be no emergency, no paramedics, and no coroner. The family wants an autopsy and will pay for it. We wish to donate his brain to science. I know dad wouldn't want to be resuscitated."

Debbie signed the consents and I gave her copies of all the documents. She knew that at any time she could revoke or take Ernie off hospice, and likewise hospice could discharge Ernie if his condition improved making him no longer hospice appropriate.

With a big burden lifted, Debbie hugged me good-bye and left to spend time with her parents back in room thirty-eight.

To complete the admission I went back to the nurses' station, made copies of the hospice consents, and placed them into Ernie's chart. I remembered to place a bright orange hospice sticker on the front of his chart and on the binding for everyone to see.

Finding Ernie was always a challenge. He could be in a closet, a bathroom, the craft room, the snack shack, or even in bed with another resident.

Alzheimer residents can hide their own Easter eggs or wake up with a new spouse every morning!

One day I found him in friend's room. She was lying in bed and he was sitting beside her talking meaningless words.

Ernie was always willing to please everyone with a smile. He would pucker his bottom lip and cry whenever I sat beside him and held his hand. The staff said it was because he was sensitive to anyone who would take time to sit with him and hold his hand.

Everyone needs physical touch. I guess that's why I love hospice so much.

My visits always included reading and singing. He never knew who he was, where he was, or anyone by their name. He would get lost and wander into other people's rooms and take their belongings, which they had probably taken from him or someone else. He could draw childlike pictures of elephants and flies. It seemed like neural cobwebs filled the memory center of his brain.

Did he have this gene at birth, did he eat too much gluten, or is it by chance? Maybe in time we will find out.

Familiar music seemed to awaken his fading memory. When I sang with him, Ernie would try to sing the words of the songs. He would always mouth some of the words as I sang *Happy Birthday to You*, *Row, Row, Row Your Boat*, and the chorus to *God Bless America*. The music compartment of the brain was still responsive, recognizing early musical memories.

The average decline of Alzheimer's disease is ten to fifteen years before death. It steals all reality from the patients. They eventually cannot recognize family or friends. The family becomes frustrated, discouraged, and even angry during and after visiting their loved ones. They

126

cannot share common knowledge and memories. Often family members stop visiting realizing they would not remember the visit.

There are ways to effectively communicate. Alzheimer patients respond to music, poetry, art, touch, and emotions. When the family member successfully use one of these right sided brain activities, there is less stress and more satisfaction in visiting a loved one.

More than five million people in the United States have Alzheimer's disease. It is the sixth leading cause of death. The Alzheimer's Association estimates the cost to care for Alzheimer patients in the United States to be over two hundred twenty-six billion dollars a year. There is no known cause or cure.

The hospice interdisciplinary team (IDT) discussed Ernie's declining status at their weekly meetings. He required increased pain medication and needed more sedation and oxygen for his shortness of breath.

After three months, the IDT evaluated his decline and decided to re-certify him for the second certification period of three months.

During the second certification period Ernie traded his voice for a weak whisper. His condition declined causing a problem with his gait and balance. He eventually lost his balance and when he tried to stand, he had numerous falls which caused multiple skin tears and bruises from head to toe.

He had one hospice emergency room visit to repair a laceration on his forehead when he fell and hit the wall. It took fourteen black silk stitches to put 'Humpty back together again.'

He tried to pull his stitches out. I made a white gauze turban for his head to keep his hands away from the stitches. After seven days I removed his stitches and turban. For him it meant time to party or at least scratch his head!

Soon the staff focused on keeping him safe in a wheel chair. Ernie did not understand the consequences of getting out of his wheelchair. When he tried to get out of his wheelchair, he fell and hurt himself.

Hospice equipped his wheel chair and bed with sensing devices that would sound an alarm when Ernie left either one of them. The aids would sprint to Ernie when his alarm sounded to try to prevent another fall. The rules of the facility did not permit the staff to use a Posey belt to secure him in his wheelchair or use side rails on his bed.

Patients have strangled in side rails and restraints. A catch 22!

The facility contacted hospice every time he fell. It required a nurse to come to the facility, night or day, to assess the injury. She would start wound care from his physician's standing orders.

Ernie always wanted to visit his rose garden. He would maneuver his wheelchair to the sliding glass door in front of the rose garden and wait until a staff member had time to wheel him into the garden and sit with him. He loved to pick yellow roses for the staff and would sit in front of the angel statues enjoying the sunshine. I would take Ernie to the garden for my nursing visits. I always cut a rose bud for him with my nursing scissors. It was there I would sing the familiar song *In the Garden*. It always brought tears to his eyes. He seemed to respond to these words:

I come to the garden alone,
While the dew is still on the roses,
And the voice I hear falling on my ear,
The Son of God discloses,

And He walks with me and he talks with me.
And he tells me I am his own.
And the joy we share as we tarry there,
None other has ever known."

Sweet Ernie would mouth some of the words through his tears. He loved music and I loved singing to him.

Somewhere deep in his soul he remembered that beautiful garden hymn. Where did he learn it?

During the second period Ernie lost four pounds. He became confused and agitated. The IDT again re-certified him, which was for the third period lasting only thirty days.

In his third certification period he became too weak to transfer from wheelchair to his bed. He could not bear his own weight. He stayed in his bed with pillows on each side to keep him from falling.

I would visit his rose garden, pick him a yellow rose, and put it in his plastic red vase on his dresser. He would smile and a tear would run down his wonderful wrinkled face. I was communicating with his heart. His heart was sensitive and full of love trapped in a body without words.

I'm never ashamed to cry tears of sadness or joy. It's always my heart talking. My left eye leaks first. Am I the only one?

It was during this last month the facility separated Ernie and Thelma. The facility moved Thelma to another room. They placed Ernie in a smaller room, accessible only to the staff.

Thelma could not understand why he was sick and why she could not eat with him in the dining room. When I came to visit Ernie, Thelma would greet me at the door and ask, "Where's Ernie? Can you find him for me?"

I would hug her, take her hand, and walk her through the locked double doors to Ernie's room. "Thelma, Ernie doesn't feel good today. He needs special care in his new room."

Thelma would scold Ernie. "Ernie, you're not sick. We need to go for a motorcycle ride tonight." She would sit by him for a few minutes, leave the room, and join her other friends outside the locked doors.

The staff told me Thelma would peer through the windows while knocking on the locked doors several times a day shouting, "Where's Ernie?"

It was during my regular working hours when the facility contacted hospice regarding Ernie's death. I received the call and drove immediately to the Rose Garden.

Debbie was sitting beside her dad holding his hand waiting to talk to me. I entered quietly, leaned down, and kissed her on the forehead. "I love you. I'm so sorry your dad has passed." I sat down in Ernie's big black papa Lazy Boy chair for the last time.

"Karen, I was here this morning and visited both of them. Dad seemed agitated and his breathing was different. The staff told me he was getting closer to heaven. I know dad was not a practicing Catholic, but I felt he would have asked for the Sacrament of the Sick. I called your hospice office and talked to the chaplain. He contacted the priest and the chaplain called me back. He asked me to wait until the priest arrived."

"Good, you did the right thing."

"I was here when dad received the Sacrament of the Sick. Because of dad's condition the priest was unable to administer the Sacrament of Penance and Holy Communion. He prayed for him and asked for a special blessing on his soul, I think he sprinkled him with holy water."

"It made me feel better. I wish dad could have understood. I left the facility for lunch. Dad died while I was gone. I probably should have stayed with him."

Leaning forward I placed my hands on her knee and looked in her tearful eyes. "You did the right thing. He wouldn't have wanted you to be hungry."

We sat still for a long time looking at the pictures she had placed on the wall. She looked at me and said, "It was a long confusing existence for dad. He spent such a long time in his cocoon. His death has released him like a

130

butterfly. I'm happy for him. I've missed my dad for so long." There was a long silent pause. "Now I can think about the dad I knew instead of the confused child I worried about night and day. I'll try to remember him the way he used to be."

Debbie began to cry. I stood up from the Lazy Boy, gave her a Kleenex, put my arms around her, and cried. "It's okay to cry. It's your heart talking. Remember, part of you left with him. That's why it hurts so much."

She looked at me with her tear stained face. "Thank you. But now I don't know how to tell mom."

I whispered, "When you're ready, let's go find her and tell her together."

Debbie and I found her in her room rocking in her brown leather chair. I gave Thelma a big hug. Debbie and I sat on her bed leaving a spot for Thelma between us. "Thelma, come here and sit with us. We have something to tell you."

Thelma stood, walked over, and sat between us, obedient as a child.

"Thelma, how are you feeling?"

"I'm fine, but Ernie's is not talking to me. We can't go shopping anymore."

We sat holding Thelma's hands. I nodded at Debbie to take the lead. "Mom, dad's gone." Debbie started to cry. "He died today and went to heaven ... He's feeling better now ... I think he's probably dancing with angels in a garden, a beautiful garden full of yellow roses. What do you think mom?"

Yellow roses are symbolic of friendship. Ernie was everybody's friend!

It seemed Thelma did not understand what Debbie was telling her. She did not cry or show any feelings of emotion. She said, "I told Ernie we should go to the races." She looked confused, had no questions, and did not ask to see him. She left the room wandering off towards the locked double doors to find her way back to her friends in the lobby.

I turned to Debbie. "Do you need more time with your dad or is it time to call the mortuary?"

"How long does it take for them to arrive?"

"They will come within the hour."

With tears in her eyes she said, "You can call the mortuary and I'll go stay with mom. Please remember we want an autopsy. I'll call the number to donate his brain to research."

Before Ernie's body left the Rose Garden, several staff members came into his room with tearful eyes. They brought red and yellow roses from his garden to tell him good-bye. They laid them on his chest.

Everyone will miss Ernie. They have lost a kind and gentle friend.

He was a favorite patient. He loved quiet time in the roses with statues of angels.

Alzheimer's disease caged Ernie in a world of confusion. Now he is free.

On days when I visited other hospice patients in the Rose Garden, Thelma often recognized me. She would hold out her arms and run to me asking, "Where's Ernie? Where's Ernie?"

"Ernie's in heaven. I think he's watching over you now." I would smile and give her a big hug, the language Thelma understood best.

I knew Thelma, being an Alzheimer's patient, would never understand the answer to her empty question, "Where's Ernie?"

Will I be taking care of Thelma someday soon? Maybe

> "I number your wanderings
> and collect your tears in a bottle."
> (Psalms 56:8)

DO NOT ASK ME TO REMEMBER
A Poem about Alzheimer's
Author Unknown

Do not ask me to remember,
Don't try to make me understand.
Let me rest and know you're with me,
Kiss my cheek and hold my hand.

I'm confused beyond your concept.
I am sad and sick and lost.
All I know is that I need you
To be with me at all cost.

Do not lose your patience with me.
Do not scold or curse or cry.
I can't help the way I'm acting,
Can't be different though I try.

Just remember that I need you,
The best of me is gone.
Please don't fail to stand beside me,
Love me 'til my life is done.

GOD'S GARDEN
Karen Farr
2015

Human life began in a garden,
In God's image to rule land and sea.
Naming all the animals
Not eating from the good and evil tree.
Adam and Eve failed the test,
Just like you and me

God told us to love Him
With our hearts, soul, and mind
To treat others gently,
Trustworthy and kind.

In God's garden of life,
It's fragile, and needs much prayer
So never take it for granted
God is the one who put you there.

Living life praising God's Glory
Loving each neighbor you meet
Telling God's plan of Salvation
Until you walk on God's golden street.

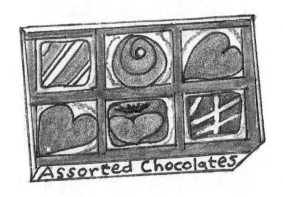

Assorted Chocolates

I WANT CHOCOLATE AT MY MEMORIAL!

Somewhere I heard it through the grapevine, this patient had chocolate on her bedside table in the rehab unit. My kind of lady!

The hospice referral started in a discharge planning meeting in a local rehabilitation facility. Alice's doctor was discharging her to the daughter's home. Sharon was present in the meeting with her mother. Due to a complication with the release of Alice, the hospital requested the presence of our hospice medical social worker.

Alice's diagnosis of end stage heart and renal failure qualified her for hospice. Our social worker asked the doctor to fax an admit order to our office.

The following day, I found myself hot and sweaty on the black leather seats of my red Mustang convertible with our social worker squinting at her paperwork. We were driving to our next hospice admit. It was sizzling hot with the sun beating on the white cracked canvas top and I was wearing my red framed sunglasses.

"This should be a real interesting meeting," Linda began. "You should have been in that rehab meeting. I'm not sure this patient will be interested in hospice. I hope your presentation will be convincing. The state mandated the patient to have a twenty-four hour caregiver. She is not happy. I've heard you can sell ice to an Eskimo. Let's see if you can sell hospice to an unhappy ninety four year old woman named Alice."

"What do you think I should emphasize during this admit?"

"Maybe focus on the services we can provide for her daughter. Her daughter's name is Sharon."

My Mustang pulled along the curb in front of Sharon's beautiful home. "Alice said she feels she will be a burden living with her daughter. Sharon will have four people to feed instead of two and she is a busy lady."

"Mmm, food for thought ... I forgot to eat breakfast."

Sharon recognized Linda at the door. She smiled and graciously invited us into her home. She gave Linda a hug. "Sharon, this is our nurse, Karen. I've not had time to brief her on Alice. We may have to repeat some of the information we covered at the discharge meeting."

"I hope it won't be too disturbing to your mom. You know, she was quite upset at the meeting."

"Yes, I remember. Mom's waiting for us at the dining room table. Let's join her."

We sat around a formal linen covered dining room table. Sharon poured freshly brewed coffee into our Starbuck glass mugs, kissed Alice on the forehead, and took her place in the chair beside her.

Is it Starbuck's coffee? I know the taste of those beans.

"Mom, this is Karen, a hospice nurse. She is here to tell us about hospice. Your doctor asked her to come today."

"Hi, Karen. I'm not sure I need hospice, but I'll listen anyway."

"Alice ..." I paused to take a sip of coffee.

It tastes like Starbuck's coffee.

"How do you keep your hair in such a gorgeous platinum silver color? It's so pretty."

136

Alice placed her elbows on the table, cradled her waddled chin in her hands, and leaned forward. "Well, I don't color it. It's natural. I visit my hair dresser every Friday for a wash, set and styling. Sometimes I get a permanent. Most important, while I'm there, I catch up on what's happening in the world by reading their Hollywood gossip magazines."

There was a pause. I noticed Linda was being very quiet. She was looking at me and nodding her head. I took the clue. "I understand you recently were released from a rehabilitation unit. Why were you there?"

"That's a long story. Do you want it from the beginning, or in a few words?"

"I really would like to hear the whole story. Why don't you start from the beginning?"

"Well, I had come back from the Dollar store. I think I had three bags of groceries when I entered the house. My key was in my hand. I closed the front door, pushed the garage door button, and started heading for the kitchen. Apparently, I lost my balance and fell. I landed on the floor and my groceries flew all over. I knew I had to get help so I started to crawl to the telephone. That's all I remember. I must have passed out."

Sharon reached over and placed both her hands on her mom's hand. "Mom, you should have been wearing a medic-alert button. All of us knew how important it was for you to wear one."

Sharon looked at me ready to explode. "We asked her over and over to wear one. But it upset her. I remember her pointing at us with her long index finger and threatening us, saying, 'Anyone who buys that button for me will be taken off my will! I will never wear it! In fact I will throw it in the trash can!' So when mom fell she didn't have a medic-alert."

"Sharon, I think I lost consciousness so quickly that I probably wouldn't have had the time to push the button. Maybe I thought I was crawling to the telephone. I don't remember."

"That's not all of the story. I had been calling you every day to check on you. Remember what you told me?"

"Yes. The only reason you were calling me was to see if I were dead or alive. I remember telling you to stop calling me every day. I felt I was okay without you calling so often. I never expected I would fall and pass out."

"Well you did." Sharon turned towards us. "And because she had told me not to call her, I didn't for two days." She turned back to Alice. "Mom, you laid on the floor for almost forty-eight hours. When I finally called, there was no answer." She turned back to us. "So I immediately drove the ten minutes to her house. Mom didn't respond to the doorbell."

"How did you get in?" asked Linda.

"I have a key to mom's house. I tried to use my key to open the front door but I couldn't. Mom's body was blocking the door. I went through the side door and found her face down, unconscious on the hard entry way floor, with groceries everywhere. There were puddles of chocolate ice cream with nuts all over the floor. I shouted her name, even shook her shoulders, but no response. I thought she was dead."

"In a panic I called nine-one-one. Then I noticed she was still breathing. Within a few minutes the paramedics arrived and rushed mom to the closest ER."

"What was her diagnosis?" I asked.

"She was admitted with a stroke. The MRI showed bleeding in her brain. They called it a sub-something bleed."

"Was it a subarachnoid bleed?"

"Maybe ... something like that. To our surprise they also found a large and deep draining bed sore on her tail bone."

"What caused her sore?"

"Mom spent most of her time sitting in her favorite chair watching TV and playing Solitaire. That probably caused the sore."

"She had told us that her chair was uncomfortable so my younger sister and I joined mom in choosing a new softer Lazy Boy. Apparently it didn't help the pain, but mom wouldn't tell us she was still hurting. Mom didn't tell us about the stains in her underwear, either."

"Maybe she couldn't see them. I am sure she didn't want to disappoint you and make you feel like you bought the wrong chair," said Linda who seemed to understand Alice's predicament.

"That's not all." Sharon began to stare at Linda. "When a social worker was informed of mom's sore, and she lived alone, she accused us of adult abuse. She reported the incident to the state health department. She lectured us about adult abuse. She told us, 'It's only sensible for a senior adult living alone to have a medic-alert button,' as if I didn't know that. I really tried. She even said, 'Even poor people can get reimbursement for a medic-alert.'"

Mom interrupted Sharon. "I was shocked when the state intervened and threatened to formally charge Sharon and my other children of adult abuse. The only thing that saved them from formal charges was my annual physical. I had that physical a few weeks before my fall. My regular doctor hadn't found the bed sore either. Therefore, the state would be required to charge the family with adult abuse and the doctor with malpractice. They didn't want to do that!"

Sweep it under the rug ... Pretend it didn't happen.

Sharon interrupted. "We got off with only a warning and the requirement mom could no longer live alone. She was mandated by the state to have a twenty-four hour caregiver when she returned home."

"Wait, wait!" Alice was raising her voice and hands in the air. "I didn't want to bother anyone with my problems. My kids are all so busy. That's why I didn't tell you about the sore."

Alice continued. "I wasn't in the hospital long and they transferred me to the rehab unit. I received good nursing care. But they made me work hard walking and climbing stairs whether I liked it or not. And I hated it! When they released me, they told me I was stronger, not thinner. It took five long

139

weeks of pain and torture to regain my mobility. That's what PT stands for, pain and torture."

"They changed my bed sore twice a day. Yuk! I could smell it."

"I'm happy to be living with Sharon and her husband. I've hired Emma to help me twenty-four hours a day, like the state required!"

"What more can you ask for?"

"Well, I would rather live in my own house, but I got voted down by my five kids!"

After discussing the pros and cons, I began the admission process for Alice.

"All that care in the home might be a big help for Sharon. I'm not sure how it will help me. I've got my own caregiver."

Linda remained at the table and guided Alice through the consent forms. Sharon gave me a tour of her home as I assessed safety issues for Alice. She introduced me to her paid caregiver, Emma, who sat on the comfy couch in the den.

"Sharon, would it be possible to gather all the prescription and supplement bottles so I could complete Alice's medication profile."

"Of course," she replied. We went to the kitchen to gather the medications out of a huge bowl she kept on the kitchen counter. I sat down at the kitchen table and took out a hospice folder for Alice.

As I started the medication profile, Sharon placed the pill bottles in front of me. I started listing the meds on the profile.

When the medication list was almost completed, Linda and Alice walked from the dining room to the kitchen. Alice seemed out of breath from that short walk.

"Sit down and relax for a minute while I finish copying a few more prescriptions.

"Be glad to! ..."

Now that's finished. Fifteen different pills to swallow. Wow! Does she take all these meds?

Alice weighed about one hundred eighty pounds and was probably five foot two inches tall. Her clothes told the story. She had not been losing weight.

Alice is an exception. Patients usually experience significant weight loss without dieting due to a loss of appetite.

"There, that's a lot of meds. ... Alice, how are you feeling?"

"Well, I am really tired most of the time. When I stand up, I get very dizzy. I think being in rehab and all that exercising wore me out."

"Let me check your vital signs and then I'll check your skin."

She has an abnormally low blood pressure reading of eighty over forty, a heart rate of forty-six, respirations of twenty-two per minute, and no fever.

"Well what is it?"

"Your blood pressure is eighty over forty and your pulse is only forty six. That's a low blood pressure and slow heart rate. Have you always had low blood pressure?"

"No, it's always been high."

I turned and looked at her medication profile. She was taking three blood pressure medications, all at the same time. "No wonder you are feeling tired."

"What's that mean?"

"Your blood pressure medication can cause you to feel tired. It means I need to call your doctor and get an order to change your meds today."

The skin assessment revealed no red pressure sores or open wounds. "Your tailbone sore has completely healed. That's good news!"

Let's try and keep it that way. What happened to that new Lazy Boy chair?

Her skin was dry and her legs and feet were edematous (an excessive accumulation of serious fluid in tissue spaces). The skin appeared shiny on her lower legs and feet were stretched tight around her four plus pitting edema, almost to the weeping stage. She was unable to wear shoes and was wearing hospital non-skid socks.

They are more dangerous than bare feet. I guess they keep her feet warm.

The sound of her heart was normal but I could hear rales in her right and left mid lower lobes.

Three blood pressure meds, short of breath with activity, probably a weak heart.

"How long have you had swelling in your feet and ankles?"

"I've had this swelling for a long time, maybe two years or more. I always tell the doctor I was born with big legs and he believes me."

She probably has angel legs, strong sturdy ankles like mine! No visible ankle bones ...

"I think the doctor gave me a water pill. Did you find one?"

"Yes. You're taking Lasix which is a diuretic. It takes the extra fluid out of your body. I think you need a larger dose."

"How much water are you drinking a day?"

"I never drink water. It doesn't taste good. I drink instant Folger's coffee and orange juice in the mornings and ice tea during the day, if I'm thirsty."

"It's important to drink enough water to keep from being thirsty. When you're thirsty, it's too late. You're already dehydrated."

Believe it or not, we're about sixty five per cent water.

"I suggest you squeeze a little lemon juice into your water. It would make it taste refreshing. Keep a glass of ice lemon water by your chair during the day and by your bedside at night. Pretty straws make it more fun and you can add a little Stevia if you like lemonade."

"I'll try to remember that."

"Let me call your doctor to let him know you have been admitted to hospice. I'll tell him about your low blood pressure, slow heart rate, and swelling. He'll give me new orders." I called the office and left a message for him to call me back.

My final instructions were to call the hospice number for any problems night or day, and never call nine-one-one. I gave them a magnet for the refrigerator and put a big orange sticker on each of their phones.

As I was leaving Sharon hugged me. "Karen, I feel a hundred pounds lighter. Since mom has arrived I have been feeling a lot of stress. You have taken the burden of all the responsibilities off my shoulders. Thank you."

"You're welcome. Expect a call from me as soon as I hear from the doctor. Is there a preference as to which two days you would like me to visit?"

"I would like to have Tuesdays and Fridays. If it were in the late afternoon, around four, I might even be home."

"That'll be perfect."

On the way back to the office the doctor called. I asked him to wait while I pulled over to the side of the road. I turned into a Target parking lot.

"I'm stopped now. I just finished admitting Alice." I told him her blood pressure, pulse, and four plus edema.

He ordered to gradually stop all the blood pressure medications. "Stop atenolol and Norvasc. Increase her Lasix to forty milligrams twice a day, and increase KCL (potassium chloride) ten milli-equivalents by one tablet twice a day."

"We'll be giving her forty milligrams of Lasix and twenty milli-equivalents of KCL, which is two tablets twice a day. Stop Norvasc and atenolol. Is that correct?"

"Yes, that's right."

"I'll write that order and fax it to your office for your signature."

"I want a potassium level in my office by next Tuesday. Send the results to me. Please call me every week with an update as we titrate off the blood pressure medications. I look forward to working with you."

With the touch of a button on my Blackberry, I called Sharon.

"Hello."

"Sharon, hello, it's Karen, your nurse. I just talked to Alice's doctor. Do you have a pencil and paper to write these orders?"

"No, just a minute … I'm ready."

"He ordered to increase her water pill, that's the Lasix. Take two pills each morning and two pills at four pm. Also Increase her Potassium, that's the big horse pill. Take two each morning and two at four pm. You can cut the horse pills in half to make them easier to swallow. Stop the Norvasc and the Atenolol. Can you repeat that back to me?"

She repeated it perfectly.

"If Alice is steady enough to weigh her, please jot down her weight for me before you increase the Lasix and the Potassium tomorrow. You can tell me her weight on Friday. We'll have a starting point to determine how much water weight she'll lose. I'll also draw the blood sample the doctor ordered next week.

For the next few weeks, as I decreased the blood pressure medicine and increased her Lasix, Alice lost eighteen pounds. Her blood pressure and heart rate improved. Her fatigue and dizziness stopped. I could see her ankle bones!

She began to feel better. "It's almost like being my old self again. I have my energy back and I can help Sharon with some knitting and sewing. I'm going to be happy living with my daughter and her husband. I'm glad you're my nurse."

During my weekly visits, I learned Alice had lived alone without her husband for the past forty-five years. She was only forty-nine when he died leaving her with a five year old to raise and three other children still at home. Her youngest daughter did not leave the home until Alice was sixty-three. For the next thirty-one years she lived alone.

"It has its advantages you know. I could eat anything I wanted, when I wanted, and if I didn't eat all day, who really cared?"

While in her own home, she slept in one of her two twin beds, saving the other for her great granddaughter. She loved to sleep in that 'old grandma's feather' bed.

Alice reserved the spare bedroom for her married children or other grandchildren who lived too far away to visit in one day.

Living at Sharon's home, she missed her activities while living alone. She told me she had enjoyed keeping track of her neighbors' comings and goings through her front window. "I could write a book about it. I would call it 'People do the Strangest Things.'"

She was a woman of faith in God and raised her children the same way. She loved going to church every Sunday. She told me how she used to drive her widow friends to church, carting their canes and walkers in her trunk. "They're all dead now. I wonder why I'm still here."

She made meals every week for her brother-in-law after his wife passed away. She would drive the meals to his retirement home and spend time reminiscing when both their spouses had been alive. "He's dead now too. I'm the only one left behind."

When she lived in her own home, she spent time in her comfortable old blue Lazy Boy chair playing a card game called *Free Cell*. She had worn out two decks of cards. Another way to pass her long lonely hours was watching TV. She never missed an episode of *"Judge Judy."* She looked like an airplane pilot with her headphones in place, which her children had bought. She could sit happily for hours being entertained with old movies and would fall asleep watching the eleven o'clock news. "One of my sons would call me late at night, around eleven o'clock. He knew I'd be up watching the news or *Nightline* with Ted Koppel. Sometimes he was my night alarm clock to go to bed."

145

When family members visited her or when she visited with friends, she loved to play Mexican train dominoes. Her best games were with her children and grandchildren. "It helps me keep my mind active. I usually win. You know, it's a game of skill, not luck."

In confidence, she told me she marked her double zero domino with chocolate to help her win at Mexican Train.

Does Alice lick the chocolate off at the end of the games? Someday they'll catch her!

Sharon and her husband were 'early to bed and early to rise' people and Alice was turning in early with her caregiver, who slept in the same bedroom.

Alice's strong determination and quick wit left a big impression. She told me, "I'm a mix of Irish and English. That's what gave me my strong constitution!"

Did Alice have red hair when she was young? Does she have a temper? She is determined.

As I visited her for almost two years, she proved to be the hub of her family. She not only knew all her children's birthdays, but also their spouses' birthdays. Alice adored her grandchildren and great grandchildren that together numbered twenty-seven. Sharp as a tack, she still remembered to send them all birthday cards.

She had a practice of giving her children and their spouses a birthday gift each year, a certificate for one pound box of See's candy.

Next to giving chocolate, her other favorite activity was eating chocolate. She ate chocolate whenever it called her name. That meant at least twice a day. When she ran out of See's candy she substituted a Snicker's candy bar. She admitted, "Snickers are almost as good as See's candy. Chocolate chips also work pretty well, too."

"What's your favorite food?"

"Bacon every morning and lots of chocolate."

"Sounds like a balanced diet to me!"

Bacon in one hand, chocolate in the other.

146

She loved bacon and eggs, and buttered toast with a tablespoon of Knotts' Boysenberry Jam. "My eggs, bacon, jam, and candy are the reasons I am still alive. I'm not going to stop now.

"On rare occasions I have a bowl of oatmeal and raisins with tons of brown sugar."

Who can argue with that? I'm not going to suggest a healthier diet.

Why should I try to fix something that isn't broken? Hospice is allowing the patient to do as they choose as long as they are safe and comfortable! Nurses, take you nursing cap off and stay flexible!

Alice had been frugal her whole life. She had pinched her pennies and bought most of her food at the Dollar Store. Because 'less is more,' she had saved for a rainy day. It was pouring now and she needed her lifelong savings. With her savings she hired her twenty-four hour care companion, Emma.

Every day is a gift to live to its fullest. Alice enjoyed her final days with Sharon. At the end of the day there was always time for drinking a cup of tea with honey, eating a few chocolate chip cookies, and sharing the day's activities.

Having breakfast out once a month with her two daughters was at the top of her list of enjoyment. It was always her treat. They were her two special girls.

How she loved her family.

Emma was a bonded caregiver from a local nursing agency. She was available to Alice at the ring of a bell for all of her needs. When Emma needed time off, the agency would provide a substitute. This was a blessing for Sharon who felt free to remain busy in her own life of grandchildren, volunteering, and sewing.

Emma and Alice became best friends. I can still hear Alice's voice crying out, "Emma, I need you."

"Yes, Momma, be right there." Emma would appear with a smile on her face. "What do you need Momma?"

At one of my bi-weekly visits, Emma had told me Alice had fallen in the bathroom. "She fell straight backwards and landed on top of me. I broke her fall. It took me a long time to climb out from under her. When we realized neither one of us was hurt, we laughed hysterically. I couldn't get her off the floor. It happened I was able to get a neighbor to help me lift her."

Emma did not know she could have called the fire department at their non-emergency phone number. I looked up the number and placed it on the refrigerator. "Please call this number if it happens again. They will come out and pick Alice up safely, without taking a chance of hurting you or the neighbor. Don't forget the rule to call hospice every time she falls or has any accident, even if the firemen make a visit. A nurse must come out and check her for any cuts, bruises, skin tears, or serious injuries."

How many Band-Aids have I opened in a life time? Probably tens of thousands!

Emma made a 'pinky promise.' She would call the hospice number every time Alice fell or was complaining of pain.

It was time to confront Alice with my safety concerns regarding her falling. She had confided in me she had lost her balance years ago and was good at bouncing off walls. Now her balance problem needed attention. I told her I would order a walker to help as she shuffled around the house.

"I don't need a walker. I walk a little bit around the house. I don't go anywhere. I can't drive. I gave my car to my great granddaughter. I'm stuck here!"

"Your daughter can put it in the garage until you feel you need it."

"I guess I can do that."

Many times Emma called to report another fall. Entering her home, I would find Alice smiling at me saying her famous quote, "What's going on?" as if nothing had happened.

At each visit I would remind her of the walker in the garage. "You should use the walker in the garage to prevent another fall."

She would smile. "I will sometime, if I can remember!"

When I reminded the daughter to retrieve the walker from the garage, she said, "She won't use it. She's very stubborn. She is a firm believer in 'mother knows best.'"

Every member of the hospice team had the opportunity to visit with Alice as she shared her life's story, her faith in God, and his Son, Jesus. She told me, "I'm a hospice missionary. I tell all my hospice visitors how they need to believe in Jesus." She even requested a special visit with the hospice chaplain so she could tell him her view of heaven, and how he could get there!

I'd love to be a fly on the wall that day!

A leather photo album of all of her children and grandchildren was always on the coffee table. She had it ready to share with anyone who would look at the pictures and listen to her stories.

At ninety-four, she had concluded people were only interested in sharing about their families. "They never ask me about my children. They only talk about their children and their grandchildren."

During a visit, she asked if she could have a hospice volunteer every Monday. I spoke with our hospice volunteer coordinator who knew the perfect match for Alice. Lizzy was eighty years 'young.'

Alice said, "It breaks up the long weeks of waiting for heaven." She had found a friend who was faithful to see her every Monday. Lizzy bought a journal to record all the stories Alice told her. Later she gave the book of memories to Sharon.

Wouldn't it be nice if everyone considered being a hospice volunteer? It could be life changing.

"Time for me is like a snail crawling on a frosty day. Days, and especially nights, are in slow motion. My eyes can no longer see to crochet Afghans. My hearing is gone unless I

149

have my hearing aids in place. Without my glasses, I'm blind as a bat and without my hearing aids, I'm deaf as a doornail."

Alice reserved Thursdays for spending time with her lifelong friend, Laura. Both the volunteer and Laura stocked chocolates in her candy dish. What Alice did not eat herself, she kept for her family and friends.

She loves chocolate almost as much as I do.

At one of my visits, she told me about her new electric wheelchair. "My children bought me a new candy apple red motorized wheelchair. After one fast and furious ride through the neighborhood, I decided it was dangerous. It went faster than my brain. We retired it to the garage to collect dust. That was a real waste of money!"

The question surfaced regarding burial arrangements. Sharon said. "When dad died, mom purchased enough burial plots for everyone. Mom has made arrangements so all of her children can be buried together. We visit dad's grave every holiday."

Alice's legs began to weaken. Her gait became more unsteady. When she fell and cut her head, the doctor at the emergency room sewed her gaping wound together with fifteen blue nylon stitches. She signed the revocation consent form. Her former insurance carrier covered the visit.

Lucky, no concussion this time!

After the long six hour wait in ER she decided to start using her walker. It helped her navigate the long hall to her bedroom. She started spending most of her time in the family room where she enjoyed a new 'pop out' chair and trusty TV tray for her snacks. The sunshine every morning through the front windows lifted her spirits.

She started sleeping longer hours, until nine or ten in the morning."

Eventually even chocolate did not taste good. Alice started refusing to eat. She became more short of breath and stayed in bed listening to her favorite Christian radio station. All she really wanted was a Hershey chocolate malt twice a day. She refused all medications. "I can't do this anymore. I'm ready to see Jesus."

Her feet and hands were cold to touch and her finger nails appeared slightly blue. I ordered her an oxygen concentrator to relieve increasing shortness of breath and a mild sedative to relax.

It was at the beginning of her last week on earth, she shared with me a vision. "Karen, I was lying here in my bed and I saw a man in my room. He was saying to me, 'Come. Come.' He was motioning for me to come with him. Who do you think I saw?"

"Who do you think it was?"

"I thought it was my husband, but I'm not sure. It could have been Jesus. I couldn't see his face."

"Yes, it could have been, or maybe your angel."

I believe in angels appearing to humans. Long ago Angels Gabriel and Michael appeared to men as humans. I might be entertaining angels unaware.

"You may be right. Remember, it's okay if you go with him. Your family will be happy for you if you go. Don't fight to stay here."

"I'm tired of being a burden. It's time. I know I'll be leaving soon, at least I hope so. What do you think?"

Holding her hand and looking into her steel grey blue eyes I said, "You'll enjoy your flight to a much better place, where there's lots of chocolate and streets of gold. It'll happen at the right time. You'll be able to run, dance, and celebrate with your husband. You'll fly to heaven on the wings of an angel and be present with God forever."

"I'm not sure how to tell Sharon I am dying. It's so difficult to talk with my children. I feel like they're expecting me to live. My body is telling me I can't! It's not my choice. Maybe you can tell Sharon how I feel."

"I'll let Sharon know. She needs to accept the fact you will be leaving soon, even though you'd like to stay."

She looked at me with those beautiful eyes still twinkling. With a weak voice she said, "I have a special request."

"What's that?"

"I'd love to have my family come for dinner one more time. I'll pay for the pizza!"

Before I left that day I spoke with Sharon. "Your mom is getting close to leaving us. It's days now, not weeks. I'll need to make daily visits now."

"Why do you need to do that?"

"I can see a definite decline in her condition. She's almost unable to talk. She's finding it difficult to breathe even with continuous oxygen. She can't move herself in bed and is anxious. I might need to ask the doctor to adjust her medication to be sure she's comfortable. I know this is very hard for you"

"She's a strong lady. I think she'll hold on."

"Alice told me today she doesn't want to leave you, but her body will not let her stay. Can you understand that?"

"My head understands, but my heart doesn't. I don't want her to die. I love her too much to talk about death. Do you think she knows she's dying?"

"Yes. They always know first."

Saying good-bye is always hard. I had a friend who wouldn't say it. She would always say, "See you soon."

"You know, no one gets to choose life or death. Death is a reality that will happen to all of us. We can only make it easier by giving permission. Do you think you can do that?"

"I'll try. It won't be easy."

"Alice wants to have a pizza party for the family. She would like to enjoy the family one more time. She won't be able to get out of bed or eat pizza, but she will be able to see and hear everyone. Do you think you can arrange it?"

"That's a great Idea. I'll do it right away."

"Alice wants to pay for the pizza."

"That's my mom. She doesn't want to inconvenience anyone. But it won't be necessary."

"We'll have the pizza, like mom asked, and I'll make mom's favorite dessert, magic bars. I know mom would love to see everyone. Can you join us? We'd love to have you come. We consider you part of the family."

At the end of life's road it's family and friends my patients request, not more material things. I've never seen a hearse pulling a U-haul trailer!

"Alice is a special lady. I'd enjoy coming if I come as your friend, not as a hospice nurse."

"Your mom's body is shutting down, unable to function or hold her spirit. Please, let your mom know you understand. I'll be back tomorrow. I'll be here if you need me." I gave her a big hug and her embrace told me she understood.

When I returned the next day Alice was so short of breath she could barely speak. I sat down on her bed. "I talked with Sharon yesterday and shared how you felt about leaving her. Did she talk to you?"

She shook her head. "She hasn't yet." I did my nursing evaluation, sang to her, and read her favorite heaven passage in John fourteen. I took her cold hand in mine and asked if I could pray. She nodded.

We bowed our heads. "Dear God, we ask your will be done. Please help Alice's family to understand you will be taking her home soon. Comfort them as she leaves. Give courage to Sharon to speak with Alice today. Amen." I could feel Alice squeezing my hand.

It's her way of saying 'Amen.'

On the way out of the house, I saw Sharon. "Sharon, it won't be long. Have you had a chance to talk to you mom about our conversation yesterday?"

"No, I haven't. It's too hard. I can't find the right words or the right time."

"Tell her you understand she's leaving soon. Tell her you love her and will miss her. Let her know it's okay for her to find your dad."

On the following day, I started with my nursing evaluation. I took her pressure, listened to her heart and lungs, and assessed her skin. She was breathing rapidly. I noticed her edematous legs were beginning to mottle with a blue and purple pattern. She was unable to speak. "Hi Alice, It's me. I know you can't talk to me, but I know you can hear me. Your waiting is almost over and soon you will be with your husband." She gave me a faint smile. "Did Sharon talk with you about heaven and giving you permission to go?" She nodded her head and added a little smile.

I knew Sharon had talked with her and now Alice could anticipate her final journey. I kissed her on the forehead. "I'll let you rest. I love you very much. Angels may fly you home tonight. Otherwise I'll see you in the morning."

Sharon was able to arrange the pizza party in two days. All five families gathered in the living room. Alice was too weak to join them, but I know she could hear them. Each member of the family took time to sit with her and share final moments. She couldn't voice her words, but she could listen and hold their warm hands.

It was rewarding to see how much her family loved her. They had tears as they came out of her room.

Do those tears mean they understand she's really going to die? It might be the last time they'll see her? Sharon knows, Alice knows.

As I sat at the dining room table, I asked family members, "How do you feel Alice is doing?" After their comments, I told them, "It will be very soon. Be sure you say good-bye and give her permission to join her husband."

When it came time for me to leave, I sat by Alice one more time. She could barely open her eyes. I kissed her on her cheek. Before I left, I administered a few drops of Ativan under her tongue for her anxiety and sublingual morphine to keep her comfortable. "Sleep with the angels. It won't be long now. Here's my prayer for you."

Now I lay you down to sleep.
I pray the Lord your soul to keep.
If you should die before you wake,
I pray the Lord your soul to take.

Guard her Jesus, through the night,
And wake her with your morning light.

I said this prayer every night as a child kneeling with my mother and prayed it with my own five children.

"Enjoy your heaven bound flight. It will be in a twinkling of an eye. You won't need a seat belt."

Emma was sitting on her bed. "Emma, come here. I want to give you a hug from Alice." She came to me with open arms and tears streaming down her face. "You've been a wonderful nurse and faithful friend. No one could have done better. She loves you so much. Thank you."

Then I instructed her to continue the medication every two hours and call hospice if necessary.

As I left the house, I told Sharon I would be on call if she needed me. When I went out the front door, all the family had gone except for Alice's son and wife. They were spending the night because their home was a distance away.

In the morning Sharon called hospice. Alice had died. My phone rang from the answering service at about seven thirty. I remember Sharon's words. "Mom's with dad now. She met him and her Savior early this morning."

I could hear tears in her voice.

"Come when you can. I've already called the mortuary and they have taken her body away. We're okay. I'm so glad you came last night. It was a great party, wasn't it?"

"Yes. It was the party Alice wanted. It's important I come to discard the medications and give you a hug."

"You can come anytime that fits into your schedule. I'll be home. You're always welcome here."

When I arrived, Sharon told me of Alice's departure. "After the party last night my brother and his wife decided to spend the night. Emma gave Alice the Ativan and morphine at one. She set the clock for three."

"When Emma woke to give the medication at three, she noticed mom's breathing was noisy, just as you said it would happen. Mom did not respond to her touch or voice."

"Emma knocked softly on my bedroom door. She told me, 'I think Momma's leaving us soon. Would you like to be with her?'"

"I told her to wake my brother and his wife. They jumped out of bed."

"Emma had propped mom up in bed. She was making a loud noisy gurgling sound."

"My sister-in-law and I held her hands, while my brother gently rubbed her cold feet. I said, 'Mom, we'll stay with you until you see Jesus. It's okay for you to go. We know dad will be waiting to see you.'"

"Together we sang two of her favorite hymns about Jesus. After the second song, mom took her last breath. I remembered what mom had said to me. 'Don't cry for me when I'm gone. Rejoice, because I'll be in heaven waiting for you!'"

"Sharon, Alice was taken on the wings of her angel to her new home with God forever. She certainly was one of God's precious saints."

Sharon paused for a moment.

"Today is Sunday. I think I'll stay home from church and call everyone. We'll probably have the burial and memorial soon. Would you be able to attend the graveside and the memorial?"

"Yes, I'll try. Unless there is an emergency, I'll be there. Let me know the day and time."

Only the family and I attended Alice's graveside service. Each sibling shared how much their mother meant in their lives. It was on a green hillside overlooking the ocean. She was interred beside her husband.

Later that day, there was the memorial dinner at a church. We enjoyed delicious homemade tamales, cheese enchiladas, and Chile Verde tacos.

What made the dinner celebration special was the open boxes of chocolate. Sharon told me Alice had requested See's chocolate for everyone to enjoy.

I am sure there are at least forty pounds of chocolate for this celebration of Alice's life. She got what she wanted, chocolate at her memorial. Who could ever forget Alice? Not I!

Alice had made one final request regarding her celebration. "Each of my children and each of their spouses are to receive a pound of their favorite See's chocolates." Sharon gave each sibling two pounds of their favorite chocolates.

Much to my surprise Sharon had not forgotten hospice. She introduced me at the dinner and gave me a five pound box to share with everyone at the office who loved and helped Alice. I was speechless.

This is the sweetest thank you ever. The hardest part is keeping the box closed until the next team meeting!

The Scriptures speak of the death of those who have faith in God. The Psalmist calls them "saints" or faithful servants.

"Precious in the eyes of the Lord is the death of his faithful servants." Psalms 116:15 (NIV)

A NEW HEAVEN
WITH STREETS OF GOLD
John the Apostle
Revelation 21
(NEV)

And I saw a new heaven and a new earth: for the first heaven and the first earth were passed away; and there was no more sea.

And I John saw the holy city, New Jerusalem, coming down from God out of heaven, prepared as a bride adorned for her husband. And I heard a great voice out of heaven saying, "Behold, the tabernacle of God *is* with men, and he will dwell with them, and they shall be his people, and God himself shall be with them, *and be* their God. God shall wipe away all tears from their eyes; and there shall be no more death, neither sorrow, nor crying, neither shall there be any more pain: for the former things are passed away."

And he that sat upon the throne said, "Behold, I make all things new." And he said unto me, "Write: for these words are true and faithful." And he said unto me, "It is done. I am Alpha and Omega, the beginning and the end. I will give unto him that is thirsty of the fountain of the water of life freely. He that overcomes shall inherit all things; and I will be his God, and he shall be my son. But the fearful, and unbelieving, and the abominable, and murderers, and whoremongers, and sorcerers, and idolaters, and all liars, shall have their part in the lake which burns with fire and brimstone: which is the second death."

And there came unto me one of the seven angels which had the seven vials full of the seven last plagues, and talked with me, saying, "Come here, I will show you the bride, the Lamb's wife."

And he carried me away in the spirit to a great and high mountain, and showed me that great city, the holy Jerusalem, descending out of heaven from God, having the glory of God: and her light *was* like unto a stone most precious, even like a jasper stone, clear as crystal; And had a wall great and high, *and* had twelve gates, and at the gates twelve angels, and names written thereon, which are *the names* of the twelve tribes of the children of Israel: On the east three gates; on the north three gates; on the south three gates; and on the west three gates. And the wall of the city had twelve foundations, and in them the names of the twelve apostles of the Lamb.

And he that talked with me had a golden reed to measure the city, the gates, and the wall. And the city lies foursquare, and the length is as large as the width: and he measured the city with the reed, twelve thousand furlongs. The length and the breadth and the height of it are equal. And he measured the wall, a hundred *and* forty- four cubits, according to the measure of a man, that is, of the angel. And the building of the wall was of jasper: and the city was pure gold, like unto clear glass. And the foundations of the wall of the city were garnished with all manner of precious stones. The first foundation was jasper; the second, sapphire; the third, a chalcedony; the fourth, an emerald; The fifth, sardonyx; the sixth, sardius; the seventh, chrysolite; the eighth, beryl; the ninth, a topaz; the tenth, a chrysoprasus; the eleventh, a jacinth; the twelfth, an amethyst. And the twelve gates were twelve pearls; every gate was one pearl: and the street of the city was pure gold, as it were transparent glass.

And I saw no temple there: for the Lord God Almighty and the Lamb are the temple. And the city had no need of the sun, nor of the moon, to shine in it: for the glory of God lightened it, and the Lamb is the light of it. And the nations which are saved shall walk in the light of it: and the kings of the earth bring their glory and honor into it. And the gates shall not be shut at all by day: for there shall be no night there. And they shall bring the glory and honor of the nations into it. And no one shall enter into it who does abomination, or makes a lie: but only those who are written in the Lamb's book of life.

Revelation 21.

QUEEN VICTORIA

Stepping out of my air conditioned car into a one hundred degree July blast of wind and sand, I grabbed my black leather nursing bag with my hair blowing in my face. I could feel the sweat beginning to trickle down my back.

I checked the address again. It was 7177 Sunshine Lane. I was at the right house, but I could not believe what my eyes were seeing. My patient's home looked like an old medieval castle.

My feet could feel the radiating heat from the winding sidewalk as I began to navigate the narrow pathway to the massive front door. The stained glass windows stood glaring in the sunlight, causing me to squint in spite of my black rimmed sunglasses. There was some relief as I entered the shadows of the porch and climbed up four steps between two tall grey columns. The two white stone lion statues were flanking the front door as if they were protecting the house. I patted the female's paw which was resting on a ball.

Hmm, not growling today!

After a deep breath, I rang the antique silver-plated doorbell. The chimes began to sound. I felt certain someone would answer the door. After a few minutes no one appeared so I rang the bell again and tried humming the notes in my head. No response. As I reached to knock on the door, it slowly opened. There appeared a tall classy lady with a picture-perfect hairdo, immaculate makeup, and the strong scent of Chantilly Lace.

My grandmother wore that perfume.

As I peered into the house I could see why it took so long for her arrival. She had ridden down her beautiful light blue carpeted staircase in a custom-designed lift that resembled a chariot.

"You must be my nurse. I'm Victoria. Please come in."

This must be my patient, 'Queen Victoria!'

"Yes. I'm your nurse. My name's Karen. You have a beautiful home!"

She nodded in agreement and with her long slender arms motioned for me to enter. "Thank you. My husband designed my five thousand square foot home ten years ago."

As I entered, I saw a beautiful fifteen foot Christmas tree with twinkling lights through two glass doors. It stood directly under the upstairs landing. The tall tree filled the room.

"Wow! How unusual to see a Christmas tree in the summer. It's beautiful!"

From her five foot ten inch frame, she looked down at me. "Every day is Christmas. It's one of my favorite holidays. Its spirit's alive in me every day. Also, it's a good night light."

"You forgot your nursing cap!"

"I stopped wearing a nursing cap thirty years ago."

Gone are the days of white hose, white laced leather nursing shoes, and white uniforms.

"Today we wear white lab coats over our regular clothes."

"Where did you graduate?"

"UCLA School of Nursing, 1970."

"That's a long time ago. You must have a lot of experience."

"Yes I do. I have experience in intensive cardiac care, burn unit, intensive neo-natal care, and teaching child birth classes. I've been working hospice the last eight years. I saved the best 'til last."

She motioned to the staircase. "You can walk up that side and I'll ride up this side. I'll race you to the top." She sat on her chairlift, and with a push of a green button, she quickly glided up the stairs.

She looks like Peter Pan as she flies up with greatest of ease.

With a silent painful moan of my creaking knees and my nursing bag thrown over my shoulder, I grabbed the wood railing and started to mount all twenty-two carpeted steps. About half way up the staircase, I paused on the landing.

My knees hurt but I am keeping that a secret.

Victoria was already waiting at the top and smiling down. I returned my biggest smile.

Looking back down the staircase, I glanced at the floral stained glass windows of red and yellow roses encasing the door. It gave this mansion a look of elegance.

My eyes caught the illumination from the immense chandelier with rainbows emanating out of the crystal tear drops from the sun beams.

So beautiful. How does she clean it?

Reaching the balcony, I joined Victoria and walked through a set of double wooden doors into what I thought might be her bedroom. She opened her arms wide. "This is my parlor. Please, come join me on my favorite couch. I have a treat for you."

Sinking into her soft white velvet couch together, I saw fruit filled scones. She had tiny triangular croissant turkey sandwiches and strawberries. On the large oval coffee table of white marble were pink china tea cups on rosebud saucers that matched a beautiful pink china teapot. Behind them was a crystal sugar and creamer set.

Is it time for 'High Tea' in the castle? The maid should appear any minute now ...

Victoria interrupted my thoughts by lifting the tea pot in the direction of my cup. "How do you like your tea?"

"I like it black," as I lifted my cup off the saucer. "I'll save the calories for the scones. They are my favorite English treat!"

Sitting in a parlor with a hospice patient is a new experience. I could get used to having breakfast with the queen!

Victoria indiscreetly took some tubing off of the arm of the couch and placed it beside her. I turned my head so I could see.

There's a green oxygen tank. She must have been on oxygen before she came down to greet me. Does she wear it all the time?

We enjoyed the moment as we chatted about her memories. "I was living near New York City as a professional model for twenty-seven years. I was six feet tall and weighed one hundred twenty five pounds. I learned to love designer clothes, classy shoes, fine jewelry, and Coach purses. You can see, I still enjoy them."

"I think I'm shrinking. My last weight at the doctor's office was one ten."

"If I could have only stayed in New York, but I married Tom. Tom's engineering job moved us to this lonely town. There isn't anything to do here, but watch the moon and stars come out at night."

"There was no work here for me so I retired from modeling. He designed and built this house so I would be comfortable. It was his idea. This parlor is his gift to me. Do you like it?"

"Yes, it's fit for a queen."

164

This gigantic room held a king size bed covered with a purple satin bedspread and several big lacy white pillows. In the center of her bed was a silver colored Coach Designer purse. Lying against her pillow was a doll dressed like a Victorian Queen in her fur lined robe and crown of jewels.

"I collect antique dolls." Pointing to the doll on her bed, she said, "I call this one 'Elizabeth,' in honor of Queen Elizabeth. My ancestry is the United Kingdom. I am part Irish, but seventy-five per cent pure English. I am proud of my United Kingdom heritage."

"It was your cardiologist who referred you to hospice. He said you have end stage congestive heart failure. He feels you have about six months to live."

"What does he know? I have a few heart problems. Won't all these medications fix it?"

"They help with your symptoms but they won't fix it. What kind of heart problems?"

"While Tom was still alive, I had a massive heart attack. At first, I couldn't climb the stairs. Tom had my chairlift installed while I was recovering. After a long time in rehabilitation, I seemed to feel stronger. Then Tom died."

"I'm sorry to hear about Tom."

"Is there anything else your doctor is concerned about?"

"I've had a heart murmur since I was a child. I couldn't run and play like the rest of the kids. That hasn't improved. My heart has a funny rhythm. Can't remember what they call it, but it's not regular."

"Are you short of breath?"

"I've notice it more lately. I've asked the doctor to fix it. He told me I was too old to have heart surgery. He said at eighty-six years of age I might not live through open heart surgery. Instead, he put me on more medicine and oxygen. I wear it when I'm short of breath. I should put it on right now."

Leaning towards her I replied, "It's a great idea. Are you having chest pain now?"

"No. Sometimes, if I get too worried, I do. When that happens, I take one nitroglycerin pill under my tongue. That takes the pain completely away. I can take up to two more pills if I need it, but I'm supposed to wait five minutes between each pill."

"Have you considered that these symptoms may be the reason your doctor feels you have only six months?"

"He may think so, but I'm going to prove him wrong. I'm going to live another year or two. It's only a calculated guess. He has no crystal ball!"

"You're right. I've had patients who have lived past the doctor's prediction. How long do you want to live?"

"I want to live well beyond Easter"

"That's more than nine months away. That could be a realistic goal. Hospice will help manage your symptoms and support you however long you live."

"May I ask, why do you want to live until Easter?"

Victoria reached for her Bible on the end table below a blue and green tiffany stained glass lamp. "Easter is my other favorite holiday of the year. My faith in God tells me I will live beyond this death I am facing. I will be with my husband and my Savior, Jesus Christ, after I die. Here, let me show you."

She opened her Catholic Bible to the book of John and said, "Here, in the eleventh chapter and starting with verse twenty-five, Jesus said, 'I am the resurrection and the life. He that believeth in me, although he be dead, shall live. And everyone that liveth and believeth in me, shall not die, but liveth forever.' Because Jesus came back from the dead, he proved he was God. His resurrection is proof I also will live beyond this life."

"I have the hope of eternal life if I remain in God's grace. When I die, God will reunite me with my husband."

"How long were you married?"

"We were married fifty years. During that time we were unable to have children. I had finished my cardiac rehab

166

when Tom had a major stroke. He was paralyzed on his right side."

"Tom went on hospice and only lived four months. Because we had no children or relatives here, I had to hire around-the-clock nurses to care for him. That was less than a year ago. He died last January twenty-fifth."

"Do you plan to stay here while you are on hospice?"

"Yes. I plan to live here until I die."

Wherever a patient calls home is where hospice facilitates their care. 'To live every day as a good day' is my mantra. It can be in a hospital designated for hospice care, an extended care facility, a hospice house, a patient's home or even a castle. Victoria has chosen to live her remaining days inside her castle.

"Victoria, do you live alone?"

"No, I have a renter living here. His name is Nathan."

"Victoria, since you don't have any children, do you have someone who will be your caregiver, or will you be hiring nurses to help you?"

"I have a caregiver.

"You've hired someone?"

"No, I have a caregiver. It's Nathan."

"He's your renter and your caregiver?"

"Well, … it's a long story. While Tom was on hospice, he became good friends with his occupational therapist. Tom knew he was going to die. He made arrangements with Nathan to be responsible for my care. Nathan promised he would take care of me after Tom's death. I was unaware of those arrangements. I never believed Tom would die and leave me alone."

"It was at Tom's Memorial Mass that Nathan told me he had promised Tom he would take care of me. He started to telephone me weekly for emotional support. I was grateful and loved his attention. He offered to help me with errands and told me Tom had asked him to keep his old Cadillac running and he would do the same for my pink Caddy."

"I invited Nathan to drop by every Saturday to buy my groceries, to do errands, and to do chores around the house to help me maintain my independence. He has become the son I never had. I'm very grateful Tom asked him to look after me."

"A few months after Tom's death, I asked Nathan if he would be willing to live in one of my upstairs bedrooms in exchange for his help. He'd been renting an apartment and was willing to rent one of my rooms.

"Nathan must be more than a caregiver. He must be a good friend. Is he single?"

"Nathan is divorced. He has two teenage girls in high school. They are living with their mother. His living here brings him closer to his girls, they're two miles away."

"If Nathan is your caregiver, I need to talk with him. Do you have his phone number?"

"Sure, I keep it on my phone. You can use my phone. It's over on the desk."

My call to Nathan confirmed he would be her caregiver. "I'm willing to take care of her. I can't be with her twenty-four hours a day. I've employment responsibilities and can only care for her through the night and on weekends. If she needs more day supervision, we'll have to discuss it at a later time."

"Victoria, Nathan agreed he would be your caregiver. There will come a time when you will need twenty-four hour care. Nathan said that he will not be able to leave his job. You may have to hire caregivers like you did with Tom."

"Let's cross that bridge when we come to it. It will be a long time before we get there."

"After having hospice with Tom for four months, you should be familiar with the services we have to offer."

Victoria eyes lit up. "Oh yes, I know all about hospice. I think you are working for the same one that took care of Tom. You have an RN, a social worker, a home health aid ... now that's who I'm looking forward to seeing. I'd like

168

to see her every day, early in the morning. I want her to come before my cleaning lady and beautician. They come at ten."

"Our home health aide can only come up to three days a week. Usually it's only two times a week if you're not bed bound."

"Oh, I don't plan on being bed bound."

"Do you remember the social worker's visit is mandatory for admission?"

"Why a social worker? I'm not poor. I don't need welfare. I have no emotional problems. I don't think I need one."

"Do you understand the word mandatory? I don't make the rules. They're federal guidelines. I have to follow them."

"Okay, if it's mandatory. I'll agree to have a visit, only if you come with her."

"Don't forget the chaplain and the volunteers that we have."

"Is your chaplain a priest?"

"He is an interdenominational chaplain. But if you want a priest he can arrange it. Would you like to meet him?"

"I'd love to have a visit from your chaplain. I haven't attended Saint Andrews for a long time because I would have to use a walker, maybe even a wheel chair. I don't want my church friends to remember me that way. I was an active member of the local parish. Tom and I made a large donation while he was still alive. In fact, he's interred there."

She's been hiding her feelings about dying. She feels out of breath and is having difficulties walking, but she's not able to admit it. Denial is sweet.

"Did Tom have a volunteer?"

"No, he wasn't the social type. He had Nathan, his occupational therapist, and the nurses to chat with. That kept him pretty busy. And of course, he had me."

"Do you want one? You won't have the nurses and Nathan will be at work during the day. You might get lonely and enjoy having someone to talk to."

"No, I don't want a volunteer. I have plenty of friends from my church who will come and visit me if I call them. I don't want the neighbors thinking I have a bunch of new friends and visitors, they might think I'm sick. Heavens, they're watching my house all the time. I'll pass on the volunteer."

She qualifies for hospice. I'll do a physical exam and check her medications.

"It's time for me to take a closer look at you."

"That's okay. I was expecting your exam."

After taking my blood pressure cuff and stethoscope out, I checked her blood pressure. It was above normal. I heard her heart murmur. She was in a fast irregular rhythm called atrial fibrillation.

I noted swollen ankles and feet. Her toenails were of a light bluish color and ice cold. Her lungs were clear with diminished breath sounds.

Hmm, she's about five foot ten inches and weighs about one hundred pounds.

"May I unsnap your corset?"

"Is that necessary?"

"Yes. I need to examine your back."

"I guess it's okay if you have to…"

I unsnapped her corset to get a closer look at her protruding spine. She had a pressure sore from wearing the tight corset. It was a result of a scoliosis (an S curvature of the spine).

Models must go through a lot of pain wearing corsets, high heels down catwalks… Ugh. I'm glad I'm a nurse, it's usually our knees.

"You have a big open sore on your spine, about the size of a quarter but not very deep. It must hurt."

170

"It's been bothering me for about a month or two, but I can't see it. I have Nathan put a band aid on it every once in a while. It's not that bad. Besides I have to wear my corset. It supports me and keeps my back straight. It helps me look younger and fit."

"I think you need to keep the corset off so your back can heal. If you don't do something about it, it will get bigger and deeper. It could become an infected draining wound."

"I don't want to have any back problems. I'll have Nathan change my band aid every day. That should work."

I noticed several department store catalogues on Victoria's coffee table. The models were scantily dressed in Teddies. Picking up a magazine, "Victoria, look at this pretty underwear. Does your wardrobe include any of these pretty bras and matching panties?"

"Not really. They don't fit over my corset... You know, I never thought about that. But, if I didn't wear my corset I could start enjoying some pretty lingerie. I think the Neiman-Marcus catalog has a great selection. That's my favorite department store. I can order over the phone. I think I'll try going without my corset while the sore heals and order some lingerie."

"Let's start your wound care today."

Reaching into my nursing bag, I pulled out some supplies to use on her wound. It consisted of a bottle of wound cleanser, a package of sterile two by two inch gauze, two small packages of Neosporin ointment samples, a few non-adhesive dressings, a few gloves from my zip lock bag, plus a small roll of paper tape.

Wound care always begins with a trip to the bathroom where I wash my hands. This will be interesting to see...

Returning from her bathroom, I snapped on the purple non-latex gloves. I proceeded to clean the sore with the wound cleanser and patted it dry with sterile gauze while I talked with Victoria. I applied a little dab of Neosporin to the non-adhesive dressing and placed it over the wound. I secured it with paper tape and wrote the date on it.

"Here is a small bottle of wound cleanser, I'll leave with you, along with some samples of Neosporin, a few non-latex rubber gloves and non-adhesive dressings, and a roll of paper tape."

"You will need to get a tube of this antibiotic ointment at the drug store. You are responsible to buy all dressing supplies. I'll leave a note for Nathan with instructions to care for your wound. It's pretty simple. He'll understand. Tell him to call me if he has questions."

"I need to look at your medications you take every day. Where are your prescription bottles? Would they be easy for me to find?"

"They're in the middle drawer of my big desk. You'll find them laying on their sides like pencils."

"Are you on any daily supplements?"

"No, I don't believe in vitamins. What I eat is my supplements."

"Is it okay if I look at your medication bottles and list them on a medication sheet?"

"Be my guest. Keep them in order."

Looking around the room, I realized Victoria's parlor was one big multipurpose room. In addition to her bed it held a huge maple wood desk, a microwave oven, a small refrigerator, two dressers, and three reclining Lazy Boy rocking chairs.

Like she said, she had laid all her prescription bottles in the middle drawer. She had organized them from small to large. Each one had its place.

I wish she had alphabetized them like the hospital med room of 1970.

I sat in her comfortable office chair and began to list all her medications on her profile. I took one bottle out at a time, copied the label, and placed it back in the same spot. Several bottles were almost empty.

Looking at Victoria I reminded her, "Hospice will cover the cost of all the medications related to your heart, your shortness of breath, pain or anxiety prescriptions, and laxatives."

Pain medications always require a laxative. They are Siamese twins. You can't have one without the other.

"That sounds good to me. I had forgotten that part with Tom."

"We'll use your same pharmacy. Now they will deliver the medications to your front door, free of charge."

Thankfully, we use the same pharmacy as Victoria.

As I listed the medicines, I kept a list of those needing refills. I also placed a star beside the ones hospice would pay for.

"Do you fill your own pill box every week?"

"Of course, who else would do it? I have trouble seeing the name and dosage on the bottles. I can't see very well. My eyes are getting worse every day. I have macular degeneration."

"Would you like to do it for me? I remember the nurse did it for Tom."

"Yes, I would be happy to do that for you every week."

All the medications were back in the drawer in the same order. I closed the drawer. "May I use your phone to call the pharmacy?"

"Why do you need to call the pharmacy?"

"I am notifying your pharmacist you are coming onto hospice. I'll refill Lasix and your potassium chloride. I wrote the names of your refill med names on a Post-It for you. If we admit you, hospice will pay for all heart and comfort medications."

"When you get through making your refill order, let me have the phone. I want to talk with Sam. I've known him for eight years. I only do business with him. He's a really nice man."

After placing the order for refills, I asked to talk to the owner. I knew the pharmacist who was the owner of the drug store. "Sam, this is Karen. I'm at Victoria's house. She would like to talk to you."

"Is she still there? Are you in the castle?"

"Yes. It looks like she qualifies for hospice. Sam, hold on a minute." I covered the phone and looked at Victoria. "Are you going to sign onto hospice today?"

She nodded her head as she held her hand out for the phone.

"Sam, we'll cover all of today's refills. Victoria wants to talk to you."

"Okay, let me talk to her. I'm busy you know ..."

I returned to the white velvet couch. "Here's my cell phone, Victoria. Sam wants to say hello."

CHF, edema, shortness of breath, atrial-fibrillation, recent heart attack, numerous cardiac meds, incontinent... she'll qualify for a hospice admit. Now let's hope she signs the consents!

The conversation went on and on, Victoria doing the talking. I was organizing the admit consents for her... "Hope to see you soon." She hung the phone up and looked at me. "I'm glad you're using Sam for my pharmacist. He knows his stuff."

"Let me go over the hospice consents with you. I'll read them one by one and you can sign them as we go. I'll answer any questions that pertain to the consents."

One by one, Victoria placed her gigantic signature on the consent forms.

Her handwriting is larger than mine. What an extrovert she must be! Even bigger than John Hancock!

After the last consent, she looked at me with her big blue eyes. "Nature's calling. I guess my laxatives are working. Excuse me for a minute."

Victoria leaned forward and pushed herself off the couch using her arms. She walked with little wobbly steps to the bathroom.

She needs a walker. We need to get rid of the floor rug at the bathroom doorway. She's going to fall. Walker, oxygen supplies, what else?

Victoria returned very short of breath. "Are you feeling okay? You look out of breath."

"I'm having some chest pain. I'll get my oxygen. That'll take care of it. It usually helps both my breathing and chest pain. Sometimes I need my nitro pill under my tongue too."

Reaching beside the couch, I turned on her oxygen tank and placed the nasal cannula in her nose. She took a few deep breaths. "I'm starting to feel better already, like magic."

Thank God. I would hate for her to have a heart attack now.

"On a scale of one to ten, ten being the worst pain you ever had, what is your chest pain now?"

"It's about a four. It'll go away in a few more minutes."

"What was it at its worse?"

"It probably was a six."

"Does this happen every day?"

"No. I was pretty excited to meet you."

"Before I leave I will switch your oxygen bill to hospice."

"Do you need the name of the company so you can pay them? I have it in my desk."

"We won't be using your company. We have our own durable medical equipment supplier."

"I have nine tanks in the closet. This one makes ten."

"I will need the name of your oxygen company so I can call them. I will have them credit you with these tanks. Our company will come and provide you with new tanks. Hospice will start paying your oxygen bill."

"Oh, I can get the company name right off of the tank."
I jumped out of my seat and looked at the label. She was using the same company.

I'm in luck. I like it easy!

"You are using the same company we use to provide equipment. How convenient is that? I'll phone them and tell them you're on hospice. We'll take care of all of your oxygen needs starting today. We'll credit the nine tanks back to you."

"That's not necessary!"

"I'll order an oxygen concentrator, which is a small portable O2 unit. It will give you oxygen without needing to use the oxygen tanks. As long as you have electricity you will have oxygen. It condenses room air into the appropriate concentration of oxygen. Did the doctor order three liters per minute?"

"Yes, that's what I'm using."

"I'll add a walker to the order. If you need it to walk around the house, it'll be here for you. Be sure and have them adjust it for your height.

"You have an adjustable bed. Do you adjust your bed when you rest at night?"

"Yes, that's when I'm most short of breath. I raise my head up. That helps me breathe easier."

"We'll have a joint meeting soon with the social worker. I promise, I'll come with her. I'll check with her and she'll call for an appointment convenient for you."

"When I get back to the office, I'll call your cardiologist and let him know you're on hospice. You can still schedule appointments with him, if you choose."

"The last item on my agenda is to be sure your home is safe and inform you how important it is to be home when we have a scheduled visit."

I noticed the throw rug in bathroom. I must ask her to remove it.

"Your throw rug in the bathroom is dangerous. You can easily trip on it and fall. You'll need to remove it."

"I haven't fallin' yet."

"I like the word 'yet.' You will slip and fall on that throw rug. Maybe you could buy a new rug with a rubber backing."

Why are some people so attached to their throw rugs?

The adjacent room to the parlor was a mammoth bathroom with a Jacuzzi tub large enough for four people, a walk-in shower, two toilets, a bidet, and matching pink sinks. Victoria's Jacuzzi had become a storage bin for boxes of extra clothes, because she had not used it in five years. Her walk-in closet was bigger than most bedrooms. There were more than one hundred pairs of size eleven shoes, with clothes and hats to match.

Wow. 'Shop 'til you drop' must be her MO.

Except for the throw rug, all the rooms passed my safety inspection. I did have one other issue. It was her chariot. "Victoria. I noticed your chairlift has a seat belt and while you were riding up the stairs you were not using it."

"Pilots don't use seat belts in their airplanes, do they? I don't think I need it. Tom never told me to put it on. What are you trying to tell me?"

"The seat belt was designed to keep you safe. The manufacturer must have known there was a possibility that you may fall. That's why they installed it. It's important that you use it."

"If I can remember, I will. My memory isn't as good as it used to be, you know." I rolled my eyes and smiled.

"Would you like one or two visits a week? I can schedule you in between eleven and twelve. Would that be good for you?"

"I'd like two visits. Can I do Mondays and Thursdays?"

"That sounds okay. If there are any questions or concerns, please call hospice. I left our number on the base of your phone. Here's a purple hospice magnet for your refrigerator. My business card is in the hospice folder. If you have time, please read the materials in the folder."

"Can I have your personal number?"

"No, my office doesn't allow me to give out my personal number.

I gave her a big hug being careful not to touch the sore on her back. "I'm happy to have met you. I've never been in a castle. I look forward to seeing you next Monday. Have a good weekend."

I headed for my office to complete my admission paper work.

What an interesting day with a Queen named Victoria!

Monday came quickly. It was a typical visit that repeated itself many times.

We began our visit as I entered the door and we ascended the staircase.

Oh, if this staircase could only talk.

"That health aide was too big and too bossy. I want someone else to help me with my shower. She's bigger than my shower. The pads she brought me are the wrong kind."

As we entered the parlor, she pointed to an open package on the coffee table. "Don't you have pads softer than these? I don't mean to complain, but I knew you would understand."

"Let me see the package she brought you."

"Here they are." She picked them up and handed them to me.

"This is the only brand we use to supply our patients. It wasn't the aid's fault. If you can't use these, you'll need to buy your own."

"Can I give all these pads back to you?"

"No, I can't use them with other patients."

We sat on the couch. "How have you been feeling?"

"Kind of tired lately."

"How was your weekend?"

"Oh, I had a wonderful time with Nathan. We went to mass together. I had my picture taken with Father O'Malley. We had a special luncheon for all the senior members. I think Nathan finally heard about God's love. He hasn't gone to a church for a very long time. I don't think he's Catholic. I think he's mad at God."

"I'm glad you got to enjoy mass with him."

"Did you go to church?"

"Yes I did. Always the best part of my week. Have you had any more chest pain since I was here last week?"

"One time. The oxygen took it away."

"And your pain?"

"All my joints hurt every morning. I might have arthritis. It's probably from my life as a model and a Broadway ballerina. That's hard on your body, you know."

"I didn't know you were a ballerina."

"My mom enrolled me when I was five years old. I loved to dance. The Nutcracker Suite was my favorite. It's hard on your joints."

"Did you take your pain pill?"

"No, I'm not a baby."

"Have you ever taken your pain medication?"

"Only if I can't stand the pain!"

"You can always hurt as much as you like."

Victoria gave me a strange look! "Really?"

"By the way, did your refills come?"

"Yes. Would you fill my pill box? You said you'd fix my medications for me."

Picking up her hospice folder I referred to the medication list. I sorted one week's medications into her rainbow colored pill box.

It's like playing tiddlywinks.

"I want to check your back. Would that be okay?"

"Sure. It feels better without the corset. It might be healed."

"It looks better. Did Nathan change it last night?"

179

"Yes."

"Did you buy your supplies?"

"Yes, we did. They're over there on the desk in a red plastic bag."

"That's good. I'll change your dressing for you."

"There are some secretions on the dressing so you should have Nathan clean and dress it again tonight. Make it a habit to change it every night."

"Did you get your oxygen concentrator?"

"Yes, but it makes a lot of noise."

"Can you pretend it's the sound of the ocean? You can't get along without it. Sure beats pulling those oxygen tanks around, right?"

"I guess I can get used to it. The oxygen's always made my nose very dry. Is there any way to fix that?"

"Yes. I'll get you a humidifier bottle. It'll make the air moist for you. I've one in my trunk. You need to use distilled water. Do you have a bottle?"

"No. Are you kidding me? I don't iron. I haven't ironed for years. I'll have Nathan get me a bottle at the store."

Her blood pressure was one hundred forty-six over eighty-two, heart rate one hundred, still irregular. "Your lungs sound clear. Let me look at your feet."

"My feet are fine. I don't wear shoes any more. It's more comfortable to go barefoot."

"Have you been urinating a lot?"

"No, why do you ask?"

"Your feet are a little more swollen today."

"I've been keeping them on a hammock when I sit and watch TV. My doctor said it would help. But I ate a bag of Cheetos last night."

"Salt is a magnet to water. It keeps the fluid in your body. Eat less salt, and keep your feet elevated like the doctor said."

After reaching for my stethoscope, I took her blood pressure and listened to her lungs. I could hear a crackling sound in both lungs.

Is she's taking her medications every day?

"How does Nathan like living with you?"

"I think he does. After he changes my dressing, we always have a few minutes to talk at the end of the day. He's a very thoughtful man. He misses his girls. He works a ten hour day, every day, except the weekends."

"Have you eaten your lunch?"

"No. I'll have some yogurt after you leave. I'm not as hungry as I used to be. I have to force myself to eat breakfast. It's not fun to eat alone. I guess I still miss Tom."

I'll try to share lunch with her. Maybe she'd like a chicken taco next visit.

"Is this a picture of you and Tom?"

"Yes, it's a picture of us when we were young. He was a big strong handsome fisherman from Nebraska."

"Is there anything I can do for you?"

"Could you pray with me?"

"I'd love to pray with you." I reached for her slender hand and held it in mine. We both bowed our heads. "Dear God, please give Victoria your strength today. Give her peace in her heart as she lives for ..."

Victoria interrupted and started praying. "God, be with Karen on her travels. May your angels protect her. I am thankful she is my nurse and we can pray together. Amen"

"Oh, about your home health aide ... what was her name?"

"I think it was Dolores. I'm not sure."

"I'll talk with her and arrange another home health aide to visit you next Wednesday. I'll have her call to make arrangements. I'll let her know you like the early morning visits, but I can't promise it will fit into her schedule."

Victoria wanted to keep her normal schedule. She had a beautician visit her weekly and house cleaning every two

181

weeks. Once a month she would drive her pink Caddy into town to have a pedicure. She was in control of everything.

When Nathan was able to make contact with his girls, Victoria began to make short trips with him and the girls. She would use her portable tanks as she traveled on the weekends. She would get her nitroglycerin bottle from her Coach Clutch purse if she had chest pain or increased shortness of breath. She loved to shop and enjoyed having Nathan push her in the wheelchair through the stores. She enjoyed going to mass every Sunday with Nathan. She pretended he was her son and his daughters were her grand-daughters.

November came and Victoria's condition worsened. It was necessary for her to use her oxygen continuously. Her outings became fewer. She stretched her pedicure appointments to six weeks and eventually not at all.

She could not navigate her walker to her car in the garage. She gave up driving. She had driven to visit her cardiologist once since her admission. Now it was impossible. She requested to have the hospice doctor visit her. We discussed her request at the weekly team meeting. Our hospice doctor made arrangements for a visit with Victoria. She loved the attention.

At my next visit, Victoria shared her Thanksgiving Day. "We spent Thanksgiving at home. Nathan made a special trip to Boston Market for a takeout Thanksgiving meal since the girls couldn't come. They were having Thanksgiving with their mother. We enjoyed a quiet time together."

"On the following day we took the girls out for an after Thanksgiving dinner at the Prime Rib Grill. Knowing I might meet Nathan's former wife, I took Vitamin X (Xanax) to keep me relaxed. When we picked the girls up, I met her. She seemed nice, but I've heard all the war stories!"

"I treated the girls and Nathan to steak dinner, but chose a bowl of soup for myself. Before we ate, I said grace. Nathan's getting used to my prayers."

"The girls told me about their school activities, acting, cheer leading, and boys. What an interesting conversation. Teenage girls are still teenage girls!"

"When I got home I was beyond tired. I went straight to bed. Yes, I forgot to have my dressing changed."

Christmas wasn't the same this year. It was her first Christmas without Tom. She did her shopping from her catalogues. She was excited to buy gifts for her new family, but sad she could not attend any Holiday pageants. She did not have the energy to leave the house.

Walking to the bathroom was becoming a task, even with the use of her walker and oxygen. Hospice provided a bed side commode to save energy and prevent a night fall. I encouraged her to leave the angel nightlight on to guide her steps.

On my last visit before Christmas, I opened the front door and through the glass doors I saw Victoria sitting beside her walker in the Christmas tree room with her portable oxygen tank. She waved and motioned me to come and sit beside her.

Wow. I've never been in that room. How did she get that oxygen tank and walker there? It must have been her home health aide. She was here this morning. They must have planned our time together.

Entering the room I sat beside her, took her hand and together in silence we looked at the beauty of the tree. The fifteen foot tree was an artificial Balsam Hill Rockefeller Pine. There were red and white shiny ornaments of different seasonal shapes and tiny white sparkling lights. A large nativity scene sat nestled underneath the branches.

Victoria was staring at the large barn that held the shepherds, Joseph, Mary, and an empty manger. One black and white ceramic cow was staring at the empty feed trough.

"That's a beautiful nativity scene. Did you forget baby Jesus?"

"No, but he is forgotten at Christmas time, isn't he?"

"Yes, he is. Santa Claus usually takes his place."

Victoria pointed to the manger. "My baby Jesus will be there on Christmas morning, but he lives every day in my heart. I'll have Nathan place him there on Christmas Eve."

"Let's sing a Christmas carol together. Do you have a favorite one?"

"Hark the Herald Angels Sing."

"Let's sing it."

> Hark the Herald Angels Sing, Glory to the new born king.
> Peace on earth and mercy mild, God and sinners reconciled.
> Joyful all ye nations rise, join the triumph of the skies.
> With angelic hosts proclaim, Christ is born in Bethlehem.
> Hark the herald angels sing, Glory to the new born King."

She started to sing with me, but soon ran out of breath. She listened as I finished the song.

"That was beautiful. What a wonderful way to celebrate Christmas."

"I think most people miss the meaning of Christmas. It's really the birth of Jesus. Giving gifts to each other is celebrating the gift that God gave to man, the birth of his Son. That's why I call him Emmanuel, God with us."

"Do you know the Christmas carol, O Come, O Come, Emmanuel?"

"Yes, would you sing it for me?"

I began to sing.

> O come, O come, Emmanuel,
> And ransom captive Israel,
> That mourns in lonely exile here
> Until the Son of God appears.

Rejoice! Rejoice! Emmanuel
Shall come to thee, O Israel.

"The last verse in this carol talks about heaven. Do you
remember that verse?

"No, I'd love to hear it."

O Come Thou Key of David, Come,
And open wide our heavenly home;
Make safe the way that leads on high,
And close the path to misery.
Rejoice! Rejoice! Emmanuel
Shall come to thee, O Israel.

She's trying to hum with me.
"Sing it again, Karen. I love to hear you sing." I began
again, but couldn't finish.
*This is a precious moment. I love her so much. Singing
to her is making me cry. This will be her last Christmas.*
"Do you see that gift under the tree, the blue one by the
manger?"
"Yes I see it. It's beautifully wrapped with a pretty silver
bow on top."
"That's your Christmas present."
"Thank you, Victoria. How sweet of you."
Her love language is gift giving.
"Open it. Open it now! I want to see your smile when
you open it."
I slowly unwrapped it. What I saw made me cry. There
was a beautiful crystal angel. "Thank you. She'll sit at the
front of my angel collection to remind me of you."
"You have a collection?"
"Yes. I've always loved angels. I believe in them. Do
you?"
"Yes. I know they were with Tom when he left me, not
too long ago."

We left the Christmas tree and ascended the stairs to finish the visit.

On Christmas day, Nathan and the girls were there in the afternoon to celebrate. For the first time in many years there was snow on the ground giving Victoria her last white Christmas. Nathan brought a tray of cookies and made hot tea for Victoria, hot chocolate for the girls, and hot coffee for himself.

Victoria's health declined quickly. She could no longer ride her chariot to open the front door for visitors. She was only able to walk in her parlor and bathroom with a walker and a long green oxygen tube.

Our medical social worker made a visit to attach a lock box to the door handle. Only those who knew the combination could access the key and enter her home. Now she felt safe inside her castle.

Victoria insisted she place the lock box out of view so the neighbors would not suspect her house was for sale. The social worker removed the lock box from the door handle and attached it to the water faucet along the side of the castle.

I instructed the team to notify Victoria by cell phone when they arrived. She did not like front door surprises.

Victoria's husband had made all her funeral arrangements. After her Memorial Mass, the mortuary would cremate her and place her ashes with Tom. She told me her name was already inscribed on the crypt. The only thing missing was the date of her death.

During the winter months, Victoria continued to have episodes of daily chest pain and increased shortness of breath while resting. She began to realize these symptoms were precursors to leaving Nathan. Yet, she was not afraid to die because of her strong faith in God. A proverb rang true for Victoria. 'Fear knocked at the door. Faith answered. No one was there.'

It was necessary to increase my visits to three times a week to monitor her condition, manage her symptoms, and give emotional and spiritual support. She began to speak of Tom at every visit and to share her desire to be with him. She kept asking, "Why do I keep on living? How long will it be before I die? How do you die? Will it hurt?"

She kept reminding me her time on earth was short and eternity would be soon. She personalized a verse from the Bible. "Absent from the body. Present with the Lord and my husband."

We always prayed together at the end of each visit. Now our prayers were asking for patience as she learned the answers to her questions. I would sing *Be Still, My Soul.*

Be still, my soul: the Lord is on thy side;
Bear patiently the cross of grief or pain.
Leave to thy God to order and provide;
In every change He faithful will remain,
Be still, my soul: thy best, thy heavenly Friend
Through thorny ways leads to a joyful end.

Be still, my soul: the hour is hastening on
When we shall be forever with the Lord,
When disappointment, grief, and fear are gone,
Sorrow forgot, love's purest joys restored.
Be still, my soul: when change and tears are past,
All safe and blessed we shall meet at last.

Before Tom died, they had executed a Living Trust to give their house, cars, and material assets to their church. Victoria discovered the circumstances of life can change the best laid plans.

Life is what gets in the way of our plans.

While she was still alert and conscious of her surroundings, Victoria called her lawyer and requested a home visit to change her Living Trust. Because of gratitude and love for Nathan, she decided to give him her entire estate.

During a visit, she told me of her decision. She asked if someone from hospice could be with her when she met with her lawyer as a witness. I joined our medical social worker and witnessed Victoria's signature.

Victoria confided in me. "Nathan has never asked me for anything since he came into my life." She had changed her will because of her love for him. "I love Nathan. He is my son."

It was a visit in early Spring when I discovered Victoria was unable to get out of bed to use the bedside commode.

Oh no, what a mess. Her bed is soaked and she is too!

After giving her a bed bath, I change her bedding. I called the team report line and scheduled a joint meeting with Nathan and Victoria to discuss her decline. The team decided Nathan's two teenage daughters, soon to be on Spring break, could be her caregivers during the day while Nathan would continue his care through the night. Nathan would ask his parents for help.

"Karen, I knew this day would come. I'll call my parents and have them fly here. My mother is a retired nurse and has already agreed to help Victoria. My dad will join her. My parents live in Canada, but they can be here by the end of Spring break. They can live here in one of the extra bedrooms."

True to his word, they were at the castle's front door at the end the week. They found the bedroom nearest Victoria's parlor to be their room. They made soup, puddings and other healthy homemade easy to eat foods for Victoria. She enjoyed having Nathan's mother as her own private nurse. Nathan's mother was kind, capable, and soon became her friend.

She continued to be incontinent of urine and requested an indwelling Foley catheter like her husband. No wet diapers for her!

Soon Victoria was unable to get out of her soft king size bed, even with assistance. Taking care of her in the bed was too difficult for everyone. I asked Victoria if I could order a hospital bed with a pillow top mattress and bed rails. The bed would be adjustable to a height where her caregivers would be able to position her with less strain on their backs.

Victoria consented. "Let's put the bed in my front guest bedroom where Tom died. I want to enjoy the view he saw from that big front window. Bring my Coach Clutch purse with me. I like to keep it on my bed."

What could be in that purse? What could be so important beside her nitro?

Her tall frame demanded an extra-long bed. She seemed comfortable in her new room with pictures of Tom and his awards from being an aviator-engineer on the walls. On Tom's desk was a black and white picture of Victoria at six years of age. She was tall and slender with a big white bow on the top of her head.

At the end of life, Victoria is moving backwards and becoming helpless, like an infant. She came into the world wearing diapers and will go out wearing diapers. This is the cycle of life.

After one of my visits to her new room, Nathan asked, "Karen, how can you work with the dying every day? It seems so sad and emotionally draining."

"I remember what Mother Teresa said. 'Let us touch the dying, the poor, the lonely, and the unwanted according to the graces we have received and let us not be ashamed or slow to do the humble work.'"

"Nathan, everyone deserves a hand to hold while they are leaving this world for another. I am willing to be one of those hands."

"My patients bless me. It is from them I have learned how to live because they have shown me how to die. They give me more than I can ever give back to them."

"Dying is the reverse of the being born. Both are labor intensive and a bridge to new life. The dying process takes longer and is much harder to endure. It normally takes less than a day to be born, but it takes about three days to die after a patient is unable to swallow fluids."

"The care you are giving Victoria is a priceless final gift. It will be an unforgettable memory for you, your girls, and your parents."

"I'm thankful I could take care of her."

The time Nathan's parents spent with Victoria was short. Within the month she joined her beloved Tom, in glory, as she called it.

Victoria lived beyond her goal, a few weeks past Easter. She slipped from this life unexpectedly in her sleep. Her giving heart stopped.

Nathan found her without respirations and immediately called the hospice number. I was on call when I heard Nathan's voice. I knew she was gone. He said, "I'd like you to come. Victoria left us some time during the night. She loved you so much."

When I arrived, the big front door was partly ajar. I walked in and climbed those twenty-two steps for the last time. I found Nathan, his girls and parents quietly sitting around her bed. I placed my hand over her heart that had stopped beating and lungs that were finally at ease. I gently closed her eye lids and turned off the oxygen. She had a peaceful expression on her face.

Who did she see first?

Her body was cold and her warm spirit was gone.

What could I possibly say at a moment like this? With tears in my eyes I softly said, "She's free. She's with Tom now, probably dancing with the angels. I would love to be there to see her new dancing shoes."

Then I noticed the Coach Clutch purse in bed with her! Victoria had clung to the silver designer purse as Linus to his security blanket. Since she had moved into the front guest room, it was in her bed at every visit.

When it was in my way, I would put it on the desk. Nathan would always put it back beside her. Here it was sitting beside her. "Nathan, tell me about her purse. It seems like every time I visit, I find the purse in her bed. Here it is again. Why is it always there?"

He gave me a funny look. "She pointed to it every time one of you placed it on Tom's desk. I don't understand why, but I knew she wanted it with her. When she was unable to point, she would smile when I put it beside her."

Nathan took the purse from the bed and opened it. He smiled because he discovered what was so important to Victoria. He took out a wedding picture and a rosary.

How many times did she pray to remind her of Jesus and his sufferings?

"It's a wedding photo of Tom and Victoria. It's a picture when she became his queen." Nathan paused. "They had a story-book love. Now, they will never be apart!"

After making the necessary telephone calls, discarding all the medications in kitty litter, taking the lock box from the house, and giving back the key to Nathan, I waited with the family until the mortuary arrived to take her body.

While we were waiting, Nathan gave me a gift. "Open it. It's from Victoria. She asked me to give it to you after she died. She knew this day would come."

The mortuary assistants came to the door at that precise moment, so I quickly put the box in my black nursing bag and went to the open balcony. I called to the attendants, dressed in black suits, to come up the stairs to assist with Victoria. I asked the family to join me and sit around the Christmas tree while they brought Victoria down the stairs. When she safely descended the stairway, they stopped in the entry hall.

We said our good-byes as the attendants waited by the door. They rolled her through the massive front door and to their white van parked on the driveway.

Nathan returned to the Christmas tree and dimmed the lights until they were out.

The Christmas lights went out like the light went out in Victoria's beautiful blue eyes. Her soul is forever with her God.

Leaving the castle for the last time, I felt sad, but comforted. She had died in her sleep the way she told me she wanted to leave her castle.

Whenever I smell the fragrance of Chantilly Lace I will remember Victoria. At Christmas I will imagine the tall Christmas tree shimmering with white lights still twinkling.

I wish I had purchased a tiara to have placed on her head this morning. She's my Queen Victoria.

When I reached my car, I remembered the gift box. I reached in my nursing bag, pulled out the box, and opened it. There shining in the early morning sun were a pair of delicate silver angel wings held together by a golden heart. I cried again!

I lost a good friend! I will miss you. I loved you deeply.

Later that week I sent a card of thanks to Daniel for my pair of silver wings. I told him I would pin it on my lab coat to remind me of Victoria.

I lost my gold school nursing pin years ago. These wings are even more beautiful and meaningful.

On that chilly Spring morning, God's special guardian angels made a visit to the castle on the hill to guide a very special lady home to heaven, my Queen Victoria.

The Lord God is my strength, and He has made my feet like hinds feet, and makes me walk on my high places.
Habakkuk 3:19 (KJV)

For unto us a Child is born, unto us a Son is given;
And the government shall be upon His shoulder. And His
name will be called Wonderful, Counselor, Mighty God,
Everlasting Father, Prince of Peace. Isaiah 9:6 (NKJV)

ABIDE WITH ME
Henry F. Lyte
1743-1847

Abide with me: fast falls the even-tide;
The darkness deepens; Lord, with me abide:
When other helpers fail, and comforts flee,
Help of the helpless, O abide with me!

Swift to its close ebbs out life's little day;
Earth's joys grow dim, its glories pass away;
Change and decay in all around I see:
O Thou who changes not, abide with me!

I need thy presence every passing hour;
What but Thy grace can foil the tempter's power?
Who like Thyself my guide and stay can be?
Through cloud and sunshine, O abide with me!

Hold Thou Thy cross before my closing eyes;
Shine through the gloom, and point me to the skies:
Heavens morning breaks and earth's vain shadows flee:
In life, in death, O Lord, abide with me!

(Public Domain)

SAINT FRANCIS ASSISI
1181-1226 A.D.

Lord, make me an instrument of Thy peace!
Where there is hatred, let me sow love;
Where there is injury, pardon;
Where there is error, the truth;
Where there is doubt, the faith;
Where there is despair, hope;
Where there is darkness, light;
And where there is sadness, joy.

O Divine Master,
Grant that I may not so much seek
To be consoled, as to console;
To be understood, as to understand;
To be loved, as to love.

For it is in giving that we receive;
It is in pardoning that we are pardoned;
And it is in dying that we are born to eternal life

Amen

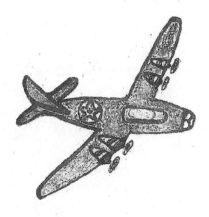

B-17 GUNNER'S FINAL FLIGHT HOME

Arriving on time at my new patient's home, I found James and Pearl waiting at their kitchen table looking out the bay window.

Pearl met me at the door before I could push the button. "You must be the hospice nurse. We've been expecting you. I'm Pearl. Please, come in."

"Hi Pearl, I'm Karen."

"Can I get you a cup of coffee or a glass of ice tea? Our tea is sweetened like they drink down South."

"Ice tea will hit the spot. Thank you."

We walked into the kitchen where James was sitting at the table. "This is my husband James."

There was an empty chair across the table from James who was wearing his orange Tennessee T-shirt. He motioned for me to sit.

"Hi James, I'm the hospice nurse."

James was quick. "Good to meet you, Ms. Karen. I'm from the South, born in Virginia. We all love sweet tea down there. I hope you'll like it."

Good hearing and memory. He can hear my name from the doorway. Pretty unusual.

Pearl placed my ice tea on the table. I took a sip. The sweetness tickled my sweet tooth and brought a smile. "I usually drink my tea black, but this sweet tea could become a habit. Thank you. It's energy delicious."

"James, tell me more about your southern roots."

"I was born on May 27th, 1916, in the same town where Thomas Jefferson was born, Shadwell, Virginia, to be exact. I was a little late to see Thomas! He came about a hundred seventy-five years before I was born."

Pearl picked up the story from there. "James was raised in Georgia by a foster family because his mom died in 1918 from the pandemic influenza. He was only one year old. It took thousands of nursing mothers. Beulah was thirty-two. It's hard for me to imagine. I was born in Kansas and didn't see death until my mom and dad died in a train accident. They were in their fifties."

"I'm so sorry about their accident."

"Yes it changed everything. I will never hurt that bad again."

My eyes turn to James. "I had two older brothers who both died with bad hearts and an older sister of a broken heart."

"A broken heart is probably the worst death."

"Yes, I felt bad for my sister."

His chart says James is eighty-four years old. His primary care physician has referred him. James' hospice diagnosis and probable cause of death will be end stage right sided heart failure.

"Have you noticed being out of breath."

"Not too much."

"Are you still walking around the house?"

"It's getting kind of hard with my feet swelling like big balloons. I can hardly fit into my shoes. Pearl has me wearing socks around the house so I don't get the carpet dirty. My swollen feet cause me to be unsteady when I walk. Pearl doesn't like me using the walls to help me. But they keep me from falling! I think it's my grimy finger prints she doesn't like."

"I want him to be more careful and not mark up the walls."

"Have you thought about using a walker or a cane?"

"Pearl doesn't think I need to use a walker. It's a lot of trouble for her to put the walker in the trunk when we travel. Banging it against the walls would not make her happy. I'm managing okay, so far."

Pearl is not recognizing his physical decline. Apparently she thinks he is strong enough to do all his activities without a walker or a cane. Denial is her way of coping with change.

"Are you able to take a shower alone?"

"I'd rather have Pearl in there with me, but she has her own shower. It's too small for both of us. I shower in my bathroom. I have a handy portable shower head."

"Are you having any pain today?"

"Yes, I have it in my right shoulder whenever I use it. I guess I hurt it playing baseball. Maybe I drove my truck too long. I always have pain in my back. We've tried everything. Even put a pain pump in my belly." He patted his belly. "It's hooked up to my back some way!"

James is suffering from right shoulder pain and severe arthritic back pain unresolved after a back operation. He has an internal intrathecal infusion pump infusing Dilaudid into his spinal fluid continuously for his chronic back pain.

It helped some, but he still lived in pain.

"I'm getting to the place where walking outside to the mailbox makes me short of breath. I'd rather be sitting in my Lazy Boy chair than laying down on the couch. It's more comfortable."

"Then you do have some shortness of breath."

"Well, yes, a little."

If he chooses hospice, I'll consider ordering him some oxygen.

"Is it hard to sleep at night?"

197

"I can't complain. I'm using a C pap mask at night to breathe easier and Pearl props me up on pillows so I feel like Humpty Dumpty. I wear that dumb oxygen mask tight around my head so I don't snore and wake her up."

"In the morning I have usually fallen off the pillows with the mask hanging over my ear. I have felt really tired lately and unable to do much around the house. I think I need more exercise, maybe a little more walking would help."

Now he's in denial!

Pearl started talking. "I have some medical background. I was a licensed RRA (Registered Record Administrator). I let the license expire. I was the head supervisor for medical records at a hospital for twelve years. I understand medical terminology."

"I think hospice will be a great help to James while he's strengthening himself. When he's stronger, we'll take him off."

"Is it true that you get free medication for your pain and a personal nurse?"

"Yes and no. Your pain medications are free, but no personal twenty-four hour nurse is available."

"James, about how much do you weigh?"

"I don't have a clue. I can't stand on our bathroom scale any more. I feel like I'll fall off."

Pearl reached over and placed her hand on James' arm. "I remember what you weighed at the last doctor's visit. You weighed one hundred fifty-eight pounds."

"Five years ago I weighed two hundred and fifty-six pounds."

"James is almost to the same size as when he entered the Air force. It must be my healthy way of cooking. When we go out to eat, James usually eats one taco at Taco Bell or a small burger at McDonald's. He's really good at watching his calories. I wish I could be self-disciplined."

Appetite is the thermometer of health. It is the first indication that something serious is wrong.

198

Taking out my yellow pad to make some notes, I asked, "What meds are you taking?"

"I take Advil, once in a while."

"I also take some heart pills." James pointed to a pill box on the table. "Look at all these pills the doctor has ordered. I'm on two heart pills, water pill, aspirin, pain pill for my shoulder, pill for my gout, and vitamins. The worst is garlic. Pearl gives it to me for my heart. I taste it in my breath when I burp!"

Pearl interrupted. "He does well at keeping track of his own medications, calls for refills at the drug store, and packs his own pill box every week. He can read without glasses, has a better memory than I do, and he only needs one hearing aid. The other ear is fine! Not too bad for an eighty-three year old."

"Tell me about your past surgeries other than your back."

"I had heart open surgery when I was seventy-two years old. They repaired five plugged heart vessels. I wouldn't do it again. My scars make me look like Frankenstein. I didn't think I'd survive. I was on a balloon pump."

"I had my gall bladder out one week before my fiftieth wedding anniversary."

"I will need to do a quick physical assessment."

"That sounds fun."

"James!"

"Do you have any skin problems like sores or open cuts?"

"No."

Pearl cut in. "He's fine. I check him for boils."

I almost laughed out loud.

"I need to check your skin for any pressure sores. Maybe we can walk to your bedroom."

Pearl followed us closely.

Maybe she's my shadow!

"May I look at your back and your tail bone?"

"No problem," as he slowly unbuckled his belt and lowered his trousers to his knees."

"Your skin looks normal. No rash or bed sores."

We walked back to the kitchen to check his vital signs and listen to his heart and lungs. His feet and ankles were three plus edema, his gait was slow, but he was able to navigate with the help of the walls and furniture.

He definitely qualifies.

After answering all their questions, they decided to sign the consents for admission. James looked at Pearl. "After all, it's free, if I give my Medicare card number and promise not to call nine-one-one."

Pearl agreed. "We can always take you off when you're feeling better."

Wouldn't it be nice if I could discharge every patient?

James refused a home health aide to help him with his personal care. He was extremely modest. He was willing to have a social worker, a chaplain, and a nurse. Pearl did not want a volunteer. "He needs to get out more. He can sit in the car if he doesn't feel like shopping with me. He should be using one of those electric carts they have at the grocery store to keep up with me. He knows how to drive it since he's driven an eighteen wheeler for ten years."

"Would you give me a tour of your house?"

"I'd rather not. I haven't had time to vacuum, get the clothes out of the dryer, or make my bed. Dad takes a lot of extra time. Remember, we had to get ready for you."

"That's okay. I'll ignore that. I really want to see where he takes his shower."

"Alright, let me go with you. Dad you stay here."

James' safety is important. Bouncing off walls ... How many times has he fallen?

James' bathroom was at the back of the house. He had a walk-in shower and wall to wall carpeting on the floor.

James could use a shower bench, shower mat, safety bar in the shower, and a hand rail to help him off the toilet.

"Pearl, these two rugs on the floor might cause James to trip and fall. It would be better to have one large slip proof bath mat to keep him from falling. I suggest a hand rail to help him get off the toilet and a safety bar in the shower. He needs a rubber mat on the floor of the shower. I'll order a shower bench for him."

Pearl objected. "We don't need that. He can sit in the shower's corner bench if we take the shampoo bottles away."

After checking the two extra bedrooms, I paused to look at the family gallery in the hallway. Pearl was proud of her family. She had all four children on the hallway gallery. She noticed my interest in her pictures. "Karen. Come into the spare bedroom where I have all sixteen grandchildren on the wall. I have a graduation picture from each one of them." She named each of them as she pointed to their graduation pictures.

Oops, I only count fifteen!

Pearl kept the spare bedrooms in immaculate condition and she had placed her own paintings on the walls. I saw a sepia colored baby picture in a large antique brown oval frame.

Is that Pearl or James as a baby? They dressed them alike in those days.

They had wall to wall carpeting in the entire house except for the kitchen. In their bedroom there was a tall king size bed with pink rosebud sheets. The bedroom looked comfortable and safe, with more grandchildren pictures on every bookshelf and dresser.

She must really love those grandkids and great grands!

Pearl's bathroom, adjacent to their bedroom, was large with a small shower stall, a high rise toilet, and a big tub.

He should use this bathroom as often as possible. It would be less walking to save energy, easier to use the toilet, and maybe he could stop and nap in their bed!

"Pearl, I hope he uses your toilet until you can get a safety bar for the other one. I'll go back to the kitchen and sit with James. Would you bring me all his prescription and supplement bottles?"

"Why do you need them?"

"We need a record of all his meds for your home folder, so every team member will know what medication he takes."

Returning to the kitchen table, I joined James. "I'm going to order you a shower bench and two portable oxygen tanks of in case you feel a little short of breath."

"That's sounds good to me. What do you think Pearl?"

"I don't think he'll need to use the bench. It'll be in the way. Does he really need the oxygen?"

"It's like this. Does a car need a spare tire? It comes in handy when you need it."

"We'll put the shower bench in the garage until he needs it. The tanks can go in the front closet. But I wouldn't know how to use the oxygen if he needed it."

"The men, who'll bring your oxygen tanks, will show you how to use them. It's not hard."

I sat down at the table and completed my visit by writing all the medication names, doses, and intervals for administration on the medication profile. I placed the back copies of the consents and medication profile in the hospice folder with a lot of information to read."

"James, your visit will be first thing in the morning. Would Monday and Thursday be okay with you?"

"Sure, that would be fine. I'll look forward to your visit. Will you start this Thursday?"

"Yes, this Thursday." I hugged him and told him good-bye. "I'll see you in three days. It'll be around nine a.m.

I'll have James for a while, probably six months plus.

On each of my visits Pearl hovered close by. She was always in the room listening to our conversations. Pearl always had stories to share.

"We've been married 57 years. I met James in Arizona when he was training in the Air Force. We were married and I moved back to Iowa while James went to war. He took our Cocker Spaniel in a duffel bag. He was run over by a truck at the base in England."

"I almost flew twenty-five missions over Germany."

202

"Honey, you had twenty-two missions over Germany before the end of the war." Pearl often added to the stories or corrected James' version.

"That was enough. Remember how I surprised you after the war? I hitch hiked all the way from New York City to Kansas. When I got there, I ran down the lane to your folk's farm house."

"I couldn't believe it was him. I about died of a heart attack. I helped James learn to farm and we stayed there for ten years. Being a farmer's wife was a hard life."

"Oh Pearl, I loved to hunt pheasants and play baseball with the farmers."

"It was a town team, not a farmer's team, James."

"Pearl got tired of the zero weather and deep piles of snow and feeding all the animals. Honey, you know you wanted to move our family out west."

"We started our own independent trucking company. I did all the book work, paid the bills and taxes. It takes a lot of work to keep a trucker on the road."

"I enjoyed driving truck, but I would have preferred farming that good old Iowa soil. I can smell it, even now!"

"Dad, you loved moving dirt and gravel in that big trailer of yours just as much. You were up at four and would be early for every job."

"I wanted to be the first one to load, Pearl. I might get an extra haul at the end of the day."

"You spent hours cleaning that old truck. You tried to make it shine. I'd rather have had you home. There was always my windows to clean, not the old truck!"

"Didn't I always get home early enough to sit with you and eat cheese and crackers before supper?"

"I don't know about the sittin' part. I was always doin' the cookin' and the cleanin' part."

"After my heart surgery the doctor advised me to retire from trucking."

"But you kept that old Peterbuilt truck."

"I kept it so I could truck with Rex if he needed me on a job."

"Your son didn't need you much. You kept washing it every week and paying to park it, remember?"

"Yeh, I remember."

"Thank heaven, you finally sold it."

"But I kept driving with Rex on local short halls! He'd let me drive his truck."

"But not very often, James! Driving an eighteen wheeler got pretty hard for you. You had to pee in a big mayonnaise jar and climb in and out of the truck with a bad back and shoulder pain."

"I remember. I finally hung it up."

"You're pretty happy, now, watching your ball games and helping me around the house."

As I continued my visits James talked about all three of his daughters and son who adored him. "My youngest girl surprised me and took me to a farm team game. We had so much fun eatin' popcorn and hot dogs. I think they won."

Often I would run into Rex on one of my visits. "Dad's my hero. I hope I can be half the dad to my children he was to me."

Their children would visit whenever they could. They were all working holding full time jobs. Pearl would say, "They never come to visit enough. I know they're busy with their own lives and our grandchildren."

James was also proud of his kids and grandkids. Pearl said he would do anything for them. I remember him saying, "There's not a bad one in the bunch. They're God's very best!"

While visiting another patient in the area, I got an urgent call reporting a sudden change in James' condition. "Pearl is frantic and needs a call from you, straight-away!"

Immediately I dialed Pearl on my Blackberry. "Something's wrong with dad. He can't stand without fainting. He's sweating and looks horrible. He's lying on the bed unable to move. Please, come immediately. I'm scared." I hung up the phone and drove directly to their home in five minutes flat.

Glad I drive a Corvette.

"If you had been any longer getting here I would have called nine-one-one."

After checking his pulse I took his blood pressure.

James has a very slow heart rate and he has no audible blood pressure. He is going in and out of consciousness. His heart rate has suddenly dropped into the twenties which is causing mental confusion.   The symptoms look like a medication error, probably a CHB.   Wish I had a cardiac monitor.

This was an emergency. He needed medical treatment immediately. I called nine-one-one.

I ran to the front closet, rolled an oxygen tank to James' side, placed the nasal cannula into his nose, draped the tubes over his ears, turned on the oxygen, and made sure the ball floated to three liters per minute. I took his hand in mine, leaned over, and whispered, "You're going to be alright. Just hold on, the paramedics are on their way."

James color looked better instantly.   His breathing improved. I squeezed his hand. "You're going to make it." Pearl was beyond frantic!

"Pearl, his color is coming back. He's going to be okay. It's a good thing the oxygen was here and you called me when you did."

Pearl is his Durable Power of Health Care. She will need to sign the Revocation Consent. I'll call our medical social worker so he can meet them at the hospital. He has all the forms.

Pulling my Blackberry out of my nursing bag, I pushed the auto buttons for the social worker, his doctor, and my supervisor to inform them of his hospitalization.

I'll put this event on the report line for the entire team later.

While I waited for the paramedics I asked Pearl, "Have there been any changes in his medications?"

"Not that I remember."

"Have you picked up any medications from the pharmacy lately?"

"His heart pills."

"Let me see his that bottle."

Pearl went to the cupboard and brought out the shoe box that held James' prescription bottles. I reached in the cupboard for his pill box and took out the next day's morning pills and laid them on the table.

She gave me the new bottle of digoxin. I poured a few of the circular white pills into my hand. I compared the medication sheet with the daily morning pills and the digoxin in my hand.

There it was! He had packed two circular white digoxin pills every morning instead of one. I noticed he had only packed one white Lasix pill instead of the two prescribed. The pills were very similar in color, shape, and size. The date on the bottle indicated he had taken the wrong dose for two days.

Digoxin slows the heart rate and strengthens the heart muscle. Too much digoxin blocks the normal sinus rhythm and it becomes a ventricular rhythm of twenty or thirty beats per minute.

He has overmedicated himself with his digoxin."

When the paramedics arrived, I told them that James had a slow heart rate and had probably overdosed on Digoxin.

The paramedics placed the EKG leads on James' chest and turned on the monitor. An EMT said, "Look at the monitor. It's showing a slow ventricular rhythm. You're right. He is in Complete Heart Block."

They switched James' O2 to their own oxygen tank and began to roll him into the ambulance.

"James, you're in good hands. Pearl will follow you to the hospital."

I hoped he heard me. I know Pearl did.

While the ambulance and Pearl were heading for the hospital, I was in my car charting the visit and calling the report line.

Later I learned the refill medication they had picked up from the drug store was from a new pharmaceutical company. The new digoxin was a round white colored pill instead of the former round yellow colored pill. The new digoxin was same shape and white color as his Lasix. The difference was in the thickness of the pill.

The ER doctor admitted James to the hospital. I called Pearl every morning to stay updated on his condition and provide emotional support.

As soon as he was stable the doctor discharged him. The following day I readmitted him back onto hospice.

He'll have to start another certification period. More paper work! We'll take down another tree. Sure would be nice if we had computers.

James and I sat at the kitchen table and went through all the consent forms. "This sure is a lot of work. I'm sorry. I recognize my pills by the color. The pharmacy changed the color of my heart pills and I didn't know it. How stupid of me."

"Don't worry. It's easy to make mistakes when they change the color or shape of your pills. Let me help you pack your medication box."

"That would be okay. Then I can do it by myself, right?"

"Of course."

"It's important to read the label on the prescription bottle three times before putting it in your pill box. This way you can be triple sure it's the right medicine, correct dose, and interval."

He smiled. "I guess I needed a pretty nurse to help me."

During the first month, James started to decline. He could no longer drive their car without getting short of breath. He started sleeping most of the day in his favorite Lazy Boy chair in the living room.

At the end of the month over a cup of coffee, James popped a question. "Do you think I could travel to my daughter's home? Pearl would like us to visit Anne. It's a twelve hour drive."

"It's possible if you feel strong enough. Only you know that!"

Pearl injected, "I'm sure he feels strong enough. He goes to Taco Bell at least three times a week. I think he would do fine traveling to Anne's house."

"Would I be able to stay on hospice?"

"Yes, you can travel and stay on hospice."

"Would you be driving?" I asked.

"No. Pearl will have to do the driving. I'll enjoy the ride. I think our Cadillac is comfortable enough. I have just the right pillow. I can sleep while she's driving. She's a good driver. Sometimes it pays to marry a younger woman!" Pearl was seven years younger than James.

"You'll need to take your oxygen with you. I'll order two additional tanks. You'll need to take frequent breaks to stretch. Be sure to spend at least one night in a motel, each way."

Pearl asked, "Does he have to use his oxygen all the time?"

"He only needs to use it if he feels short of breath, not continuously."

"I think we can do it. How do you feel, dad?"

"I can try anything once as long as I'm with you."

"Don't forget to take your medications and enough for one extra week, in case you want to stay a little longer."

On the report line, I alerted the team of James' road trip. Our hospice social worker arranged for another local hospice in her area to be aware of his visit. He prepared all the hospice paperwork and sent James' chart to their office in case they needed to make a visit. They were willing to make visits and exchange oxygen tanks if the family requested it.

Paperwork is the hardest part of this job.

James' visit with his daughter went without a glitch. He followed the doctor's orders wearing his oxygen as needed.

Anne was thrilled they had brought an extra week's worth of medications. It allowed them to visit the local National Park.

James decided to help Pearl. He asked Anne if she could drive them back home. She did.

At the end of another week she flew home. She was grateful to hospice for arranging extra time with her dad. She knew her dad's time was limited and making memories was her first priority.

A memory made is a memory saved.

On my first visit after the trip, Pearl requested I try to find a volunteer. She finally realized James could not traipse around shopping without needing oxygen. She needed time to get her hair done on Fridays and do her weekly grocery shopping.

Our volunteer coordinator chose a veteran who had also served in the Army-Air Force in World War II. They shared their war stories of flying in a few of the ninety-eight thousand bomber planes built for the war. They became good friends and the volunteer gave Pearl a needed break every Friday. Pearl appreciated the opportunity to take 'time out,' something every caregiver needs desperately.

War stories are for men who fought the war and understand the horror. No wonder they never boast about the war.

James' social worker was surprised when he made his monthly mandated visit. He found a new Cocker Spaniel puppy named Rusty to welcome him at the front door. He shared, at the weekly hospice team meeting, James had whispered this secret, "Pearl will need some company when I leave. I think Rusty will keep her busy. I call him Cowboy, but Pearl calls him Rusty, that's the color of his soft curly coat."

Rusty was content to sit at James' feet. Whenever visitors came, Rusty would run to the front door and bark. It became unnecessary to knock. Rusty was a barking doorbell!

Every week I could see James' decline. He was less interested in food, which is typical when patients are nearing the end of life. In his mind he knew he was leaving but in his heart he did not know how to tell Pearl. He told me, "Pearl is bound and determined to keep me alive. I don't know how to tell her I'm dying."

For Pearl talking about death is like having a huge elephant in a small room pressing against her while she continues to ignore it. It hurts so bad she doesn't want to talk about it. She hopes it will go away on its own.

To approach the subject, I shared this story so Pearl could understand the emotion of letting James go, whenever that day arrived.

"There was once a little boy who could not wait to go on his first overnight field trip with his friends on a big yellow school bus. His mother felt he should go on the trip. She had concerns about putting him on a bus with an unfamiliar bus driver and a bunch of kids who were headed for a faraway camp."

"When the day finally arrived, the son was excited to take the trip with his friends until he looked out the window and saw his mom. She was crying. He wanted to go on the trip, but he also wanted to stay with his mom so she wouldn't cry."

"James, are you feeling like this little boy?"

"Yes, that's exactly how I feel."

"Pearl, soon it will be time for James to go on his final trip."

We waited silently while Pearl processed her thoughts ... tears started to roll down her cheeks. She looked into James' welling eyes, "You're not going to leave me, are you?"

"I don't think I have a choice. I think I'm going to have to leave you! My body can't stay alive much longer." They took each other by the hand and cried.

Tears are like golden drops of oil. They lubricate the soul and help relieve the tension of the heart. Their tears put Pearl's denial to rest.

Another month slipped by and it was nearing time to start the tedious paperwork required for the third certification period. James was declining, but he still was walking, eating, and communicating. He was not actively dying.

Early in the morning, when I was on call, the answering service asked me to speak with Pearl.

Did James fall out of bed, have a heart attack, or is he too anxious to sleep?

Somehow, I didn't realize what the answering service was trying to tell me. Did she say 'James had died?'

"Can you repeat that? Did you say James died?"

"Yes, James died in his sleep."

I immediately called Pearl. She was crying. "Oh Karen, I can't believe he died lying right beside me. He forgot to wear his oxygen last night. What happened? He's gone."

"His heart was tired and finally stopped."

"I left our bed for a moment. After I got back in bed I felt for his hand as usual, but it was cold as ice. His breathing seemed so quiet. I tried to wake him up. He didn't respond."

"Then I knew he had left me. I can't believe it. We went out for tacos last night. He ate half of a taco and part of a vanilla shake. He walked up our hill to the neighbor's. He said he had to get in better shape for me."

"I need to call my daughters and son. They'll come and be with me as soon as they can. Meryl is a hospice nurse and I know she and her husband will come as soon as their 'Beemer' can get them here. Please don't come too soon. Wait at least two hours."

"I think I'll call my neighbor and our pastor who can be with me in a few minutes. I'm okay. You know, James really loved you and looked forward to your visits."

Tears began rolling down my cheeks. "I'm so sorry. Are you sure you're alright alone? I can be there in a few minutes."

Pearl answered with confidence in her voice, "I'm never alone. I have Rusty! He's lying beside dad. I don't think he'll leave his side for a while.

"I'll call you if I change my mind."

I called Pearl in two hours like she had requested. "You don't have to come. My kids are here and they can call the mortuary. I have everything arranged."

"James was very special to me and I would like to come for one last visit with you."

"That would be fine. Take your time. There is no hurry now. Remember what you told me? Dying on hospice is not an emergency."

When I approached the front door, it seemed strange to ring the doorbell and not hear Rusty barking. Rex answered the door and hugged me. His two sisters were seated at the bedside both holding James' hand.

It was not necessary to listen to his tired heart that refused to beat another time. He looked sound asleep, lying peacefully on his bed with his eyes closed. His soul was at peace with God.

He looks so peaceful. The smile on his face may be telling us he saw the angel that came to take him home.

Early that morning, one brave soldier returned to glory. James had shown me pictures of his B-17 bomber that had flown over Germany on twenty-two missions. He had been the lucky one to always return to the base in England. Today was his final flight. He had prepared himself for this spiritual flight through his life of faith in Jesus Christ for thirty-three years. He had flown faster than his B-17 bomber into the realms of glory on the wings of his angels.

We all dream of dying in our sleep. It seems the most peaceful way to go, but it's shocking for the family. It's more like an accident. People who experience this get the wrong perception of death. They think they will die in their sleep.

Pearl shared a special story with me. James had left his Bible open on his bedside table with his eye glasses as a book marker. He had placed the glasses in the last page in the book of Matthew. The last verse in the book of Matthew must have been the last verse that he had read before he went to sleep. James had underlined it with a ball point pen. "And lo I am with you always, even until the end of the age." (Matthew 28:20)

Pearl told me James often wondered who he would see first to welcome him through heaven's gate. She said James hoped it would be his mother.

I can visualize Beulah standing at the gate, welcoming James home. She was only able to love him at her breast for a few months before she died. Now they're home together forever.

He's in heaven where there will be a great reunion of his loved ones. It will be better than anything he has ever dreamt or imagined. The music will be more than surround sound. Every pore of his spiritual body will hear it. It will be like a thousand symphonies, too beautiful for the tongue or mind to describe. It will be in a new dimension we are unable to understand. There will be light, peace and joy forever more. The love of God will be an eternal hug.

"Eye has not seen, nor ear heard, nor has it entered into the heart of man, the things which God has prepared for those who love him." 2nd Corinthians 2:9

For I am persuaded, that neither death, nor life, nor angels, nor principalities, nor powers, nor things present, nor things to come, nor height, nor depth, nor any other creature, shall be able to separate us from the love of God, which is in Christ Jesus our Lord. 2 Corinthians 38:39 (KJV)

GONE FROM MY SIGHT
Henry Van Dyke
American clergyman, educator, and author
(1852-1933)

I am standing upon the seashore. A ship at my side spreads her white sails to the morning breeze and starts for the blue ocean.

She is an object of beauty and strength. I stand and watch her until, at length, she hangs like a speck of white cloud just where the sea and sky come to mingle with each other.

Then someone at my side says, "There. She is gone!"

"Gone where?"

Gone from my sight. That is all. She is just as large in mast and hull and spar as she was when she left my side and she is just as able to bear her load of living freight to her destined port.

Her diminished size is in me; not in her.

And just at the moment when someone at my side says, "There! She is gone!" there are other eyes watching her coming, and other voices ready to take up the glad shout: "Here she comes!"

And that is dying.

DEDICATION

I dedicate this book to all my patients, from a two pound two ounce baby boy, to a ninety-nine year old who lived to blow out one hundred candles. "You walked into my heart and blessed my life's path."

MY PRAYER FOR YOU ...

I pray this book will be helpful in your life's journey. May it teach you what hospice means and how hospice can help you or a loved one at the end of the journey.

Life is fragile, handle with prayer. Live each day as a gift. Unwrap it carefully.

ACKNOWLEDGEMENTS

The book you are holding would be a dream if not for my loving husband Bruce, who is my editor in chief, the wind beneath my wings. Thank you, sweetheart.

Thank you to my daughter, Shiloh, who inspired me to write this book. "Mom, people barely know how to live. No one knows how to die. You need to write a book. Share hospice!"

Thank you Beth Avila, my darling niece. You encouraged me and edited all my final copies. "Auntie K, keep writing!"

Thank you, Mary Delaney, for drawing the cover picture. Thank you, Carole Ross, for the chapter art drawings.

Thank you, Sandi Lehman, and the writing class students for your encouragement and guidance as I began to write the chapters in this book.

Thanks to Howard Ellowis, leader, and members of my poetry group for helping me appreciate poetry and contributing to this book.

Thank you, Marge Anselma, for your contributions in poetry.

I am grateful to hospice colleagues Randy Denham, M.S.W., M.F.C.C., and Ginny Cross Kemmerer, N.P., for your hospice expertise.

Thank you to my circle of friends who encouraged me to write about hospice.

Most important is my thanks to God who gave me life and strength to be a nurse. He is my compass in life, my anchor in the storm, and my joy in the morning.

ABOUT THE AUTHOR ...

As a child growing up in the 50's on a Nebraska farm, my mom knew I would be a nurse someday. I loved caring for the sick animals and taking care of the livestock. When I was five years old a stray dog severely bit my face. On the way to the hospital, I comforted my mother. "It will be all right momma, it will be all right." That was how she knew.

Graduating from Fullerton Community School of Nursing in 1968, I chose to work in ICU/CCU/Intensive Care Burn Unit/Intensive Care Nursery/OB at a major county hospital for my initial nursing experience.

When my family of four children became my first priority, I chose to become a nurse educator. My field of expertise became Prepared Childbirth. After receiving certification with CEALA, I taught hundreds of couples in my home how to prepare and participate together in childbirth.

When my youngest entered public schools, I returned to full time nursing. My experience qualified me for intensive care nursing including ICU, ICCU, and Neo-Natal Intensive Care for fifteen years. There I could listen to the fears and concerns of each of my patients.

I always say, "I saved the best for last." I decided to be a Hospice Nurse Case Manager for the last ten years of my nursing career. What a ride! While working in various geographical settings, from the ocean to the desert with beautiful snowy mountains in-between, I experienced the full gamut of hospice organizations: private, hospital, and government run hospices in California.

Palliative care surrounds my end of life stories sharing how hospice care supports real people whose doctors have given them the dreaded news of a life shortening illness without a cure.

Hundreds of patients have blessed me over my forty years of nursing as I became their friend and advocate through healing and dying.

KAREN FARR, RN

Made in the USA
Lexington, KY
03 January 2019